The cLEAN Mom

The cLEAN Momma Workout

GET **LEAN** WHILE YOU **CLEAN**

arnes

erk

WILLIAM MORROW

An Imprint of **HarperCollins***Publishers*

This book contains advice and information relating to health care. It is not intended to replace medical advice and should be used to supplement rather than replace regular care by your doctor. It is recommended that you seek your physician's advice before embarking on any medical program or treatment. All efforts have been made to assure the accuracy of the information contained in this book as of the date of publication. The publisher and the author disclaim liability for any medical outcomes that may occur as a result of applying the methods suggested in this book.

HarperCollins books may be purchased for educational, business, or sales promotional use. For information please write: Special Markets Department, HarperCollins Publishers, 10 East 53rd Street, New York, NY 10022.

FIRST EDITION

Designed by Richard Oriolo

All photographs © 2012 by Jan Cobb

Library of Congress Cataloging-in-Publication Data has been applied for.

ISBN 978-0-06-221115-6

13 14 15 16 17 OV/RRD 10 9 8 7 6 5 4 3 2 1

To Sophie and Jack, for keeping me true to my word and for inspiring me to be the best person I can be.

CONTENTS

PART IV cLEAN Routine

The cLEAN Momma Workout

INTRODUCTION

MOMS DO NOT HAVE IT easy—we are not only the chief cooks, bottle washers, and boo-boo kissers, we are also the glue that holds our families and our homes together. With that job comes a ton of chores, errands, and never-ending responsibility. And guess what takes a backseat while you're doing all of the above? Your life. Your waistline. Your sanity. I get it; I was in baggy sweats ('cause nothing else fit!) not that long ago. My tush was reaching epic proportions. My thighs had more jiggle than Jell-O. Why? Because I had no time to exercise after my kids were born. Not if I wanted my kids fed and my kitchen clean. There was simply not enough of me (though I certainly *felt* like I was big enough!) to go around. The baby weight was not goin' anywhere any time soon. That's when I had an epiphany: exercise and housework could cohabitate! I could clean my countertops, polish my floors, *and* tone my tush at the same time! It was like a freakin' miracle: a marriage of exercise and cleaning. I called it "Taskercise," and watched my body get back to its prebaby shape in record time. I shed fifty-plus pounds and my arms are pretty ripped for a mother of two!

And here's the best part: you can do it, too. No matter how hectic your life is, Taskercise is a one-size-fits-all solution to losing weight, toning up, and regaining your inner calm. It starts with a basic principle: you have a choice! You don't have to be frumpy, dumpy, and depressed. Your shower doesn't have to be covered in grime and your sink piled high with dishes. You don't have to eat junk food and look like you fell out of bed every day. You can choose to get your act together. You can choose to gain strength, lose the pounds, and clean up your home.

Moms are experts at multitasking. Personally, I could juggle a baby in one arm and a poop-filled diaper in the other . . . while talking on the phone and checking my e-mail. So why not vacuum your rug while you firm up your thighs? Why not unload the dishwasher as you tone your calves? It made perfect sense, and the more I did it, the more I realized how I could Taskercise both in my house and outside as well. Who needed a gym? I did leg lifts in line at the supermarket checkout. Donkey kicks while pumping gas. Bun crunches while carpooling to nursery school. Anywhere, every-where, any time, all the time. Taskercise is a simple way to sneak exercise into your schedule and squeeze your butt back into your skinny jeans. It will free up your life so you have more time to relax, to think straight, to *breathe*. I promise you, it is not only time-saving, it's life-saving. For me, it was a way to regain my pre-Momma mojo. I have never felt so strong, so fit, so confident . . . and my house is pretty damn spotless (most of the time!).

My So-Called Life

So how did I happen upon this fitness revelation? It was after midnight, in the middle of winter in L.A. in 2010, and it was freezing outside. I was standing at the edge of my pool and looking up at the star-filled sky and thinking, *What the hell? How did this become my life?*

I wasn't depressed, pissed, or overwhelmed; that was the irony. I was simply numb. The decline in the economy took a big dump on my family. Crap began to hit more than just my son's diapers. My marriage was falling apart, and I didn't want to believe any of it. I was suffering from what I like to refer to as chronic "Head Up My Butt–itis." Translation: denial, big-time. So I jumped off the edge of the pool and into the icy water. But I swam through it, from one end of the pool to the other. When I emerged on the other side, I told myself, "If I can handle this freezing water, I can handle anything!" That was my "aha moment," so to speak. The moment I knew it was time to take control, take responsibility, take the blinders off and start living, not merely just existing. It was about time . . .

I was born in New York City, and when I was four, my family moved to L.A. That being said, I always felt like a New Yorker, probably because my Brooklyn-born, Jewish-atheist mother beat it into my head. When I was six, she would make me say "cawfee" instead of "coffee." We weren't your typical all-American family. My dad was married once before my mom, so I had two half-sisters. My parents fought . . . a lot. I vividly remember looking through the banister at the top of our staircase, when I was nine, as my parents argued. My mom had completely lost it, shouting at my dad, "Let's just split the f—ing furniture!" My dad replied, angrily, under his breath, "Keep it all. But I get the backgammon table!" A month later, they divorced.

So my dad moved out and into an apartment that was a two-minute walk around the corner from our town house. Even though he remained close by, it was basically my mom and Socorro (our housekeeper/my playmate) who I grew up with. My mom was a very successful businesswoman, a pioneer in the computer indus-try. She ran the first company to offer computer-based training, while Socorro ran our home.

Because Mom traveled quite a bit, Socorro was often in charge of making sure I did my homework and cleaned my room. I had that all under control: I would copy my answers off a friend and shove my junk into my closet. School made me nuts and I thought it was a joke, probably because I had ADD, hated to read, and had trouble paying attention to anything other than boys. I did, however, love theater! I spent all my time doing school musicals, because I was a ballet bunhead from the age of five and had a set of pipes that could belt out show tunes; I was *good*!

So when it came time to apply for college, it was a no-brainer: I would major in theater and minor in dance. My mom begged me to take a "real" major, a career that might actually earn some money, but I wouldn't budge. I graduated from UC Santa Barbara with honors. Who couldn't get a 4.0 when your finals were juggling, Shakespeare on the beach, and somersaults?

After Santa Barbara, I moved into the home I grew up in with my college roommate, Michele. My mom kept the place while she lived in Malibu. She figured letting me live rent-free for a while would give me an opportunity to get myself on my feet. But I had no clue how to do that. All I knew was how to stand onstage, point my toes, and sing. So I did. I was hired and worked on show after show. That was my job. It didn't pay much, but at least it was my version of work.

In between shows, I would hang out with Michele and her boyfriend and my high school best friend, Steve. We played a married couple in our high school play *No Sex Please, We're British* senior year. Little did we suspect we'd become husband and wife for real one day.

After Steve popped the question (at a romantic château we borrowed for a month in the south of France!), we came back and shared the news with our families and Michele. We were on a road trip to visit our old stomping grounds at UCSB, and I told her that she needed to find a new place because Steve was moving in. Michele wasn't thrilled, and I felt terrible. Our drive home was tense, so I broke the tension by buying a puppy from some homeless lady off the street. A week later, I booked the national/world tour of *A Chorus Line*. I had to leave my fiancé and our new puppy, Mia, behind for six months.

Thankfully, the time flew by, and as soon as the plane landed from Korea, the last stop on the tour, I immediately dove into wedding planning. Everything moved so quickly; I never really stopped to digest it all. I was only twenty-four, and didn't understand what it meant to be starting a life with someone. I was a naïve child.

I remember our wedding day so clearly: it was a great party that took place on a cliff overlooking the ocean. We had about 250 guests, most of whom I didn't know. I felt disconnected, and a bit lonely, till my best friends found me and handed me two tequila shots, one for each hand.

The early years of our marriage were good. We were best friends, and I was doing my shows. We bought a great house in Encino. It was cute, not too big, not too small, just right for starting a family. It overlooked the park, and we had a blast living there. While my husband was becoming incredibly successful as a day trader, I continued to work in show biz, eventually making my way into TV, where I did commercials.

We had a very "Ricky-Lucy" relationship. He was in charge of all the finances. I would hand over my paychecks, and he would dole out whatever I needed to pay for things. I adored my husband. He made me feel safe and secure. He was the decision maker, the one who called all the shots. I liked that. I never felt competent with finances, so I let him take care of me. I took the easy way out.

In 2002, we decided it was time to have a baby. I gave birth to Sophie on December 26. About three and a half years later, I popped out Jack on June 20, 2006—and everything changed. The stock market went belly-up, and my husband lost his job. We grew further and further apart. My husband kept a lot to himself: not just how he was feeling but also how huge our financial losses were. There would be no more extravagant trips, no more housekeeper, no more gym membership. Yet he was afraid to tell me that. He thought it would cause me anxiety—he was still trying to be my protector. But his lack of communication caused us both a ton of stress.

I walked around in a semi-daze: I didn't know how to do a damn thing. I didn't know how to help him or myself. I had two little children: Sophie, three and a half, and Jack, my newborn. I wore stretchy pants (because I gained over sixty pounds while pregnant with Jack, and my butt couldn't fit into anything else). Because Socorro cooked all my meals and cleaned our home when I was a child, I was totally unprepared for taking care of a household by myself. I became a master at burning dinner and shrinking my husband's shirts. I hated cleaning; I hated being responsible—and I couldn't handle much more on my plate. So when my four-week-old son spit up all over the kitchen floor, it was just one more hassle to deal with. My hands were full holding him, so I used my foot to wipe up the mess. I felt the burn in my thighs. A lightbulb went off in my head . . . Taskercise was born.

Taskercise was a way for me to get a handle on the hell I was living. My messy, unkempt house became my home gym. Slowly, the weight began to melt off, and my kitchen floors sparkled! I would joke around with my mommy friends at Sophie's preschool, and say, "I've mastered the art of multitasking!" They looked at me like I was nuts, but meanwhile I was back in jeans in less than four months after Jack was born. I would tell them, "No more excuses, ladies! Do leg lifts while you do your dishes and brush your teeth!" This was how I finally figured out how to get my baby weight off, get toned up, get organized, and clean my house in the most "fantabulously" insane way.

My body was stronger and more toned than it had ever been, even when I was twenty and dancing on tour. That being said, I was still exhausted and overwhelmed. I may have been fit, but centered and balanced . . . well, that was another story. I needed to carve out more "me time." When I had my kids, it automatically became "them time," and now I was truly desperate to find balance and a system! I began to incorporate Taskercise into all aspects of my life: playtime with the kids, texting my sisters on the phone, waiting in long lines at Target. And I thought about how I could clean up the rest of my life, not just my home. How I could polish up my ego, wipe away stress, and recharge my batteries. The cLEAN Momma program was born!

My sisters encouraged me to blog about it—there were so many frazzled mommies out there who could benefit from what I'd figured out. I made a DVD showing my exercise routine and sold it (hell, I needed the money, didn't I?). The principle was simple: "Get LEAN while you cLEAN." I pooled together all my resources and got a great team of friends to help me shoot and edit. After we finally finished, one of my dear friends, Robin (she's a press agent), wrote up a press release. The media flocked to my "off-the-wall approach" to working out, and the next thing I knew, I was featured in the *L.A. Times, Parenting* magazine, *Fitness* magazine, and the *Wall Street Journal,* and I was on TV on *The Doctors, Good Morning America,* and Style TV. All this because my baby puked on my kitchen floor! Go figure!

With the help of my sisters, I was able to build my own Web site (www.clean momma.com), sell my DVD, and blog all my wacky tips and ideas. This became my full-time job, but more than that, my mission in life. I gained tons of Facebook and YouTube fans. Yet despite all the hoopla surrounding my program, finances were still tough. I didn't realize how tough till the water and power got turned off. As the economy got worse, and everyone was losing their homes and jobs, things progressively got worse for us, too. Our credit cards stopped working, and I was returning groceries for cash.

I remember borrowing $2 for gas for my fully loaded SUV (it was on the verge of being repossessed, but who knew?). My husband and I eventually split up in 2010. Today, we are really good friends and work hard to co-parent our kids. But at the time of the divorce, I felt so scared and alone. There was no way I could go to my mom for financial help. She had already helped us years ago, and I was too ashamed to ask. I needed to figure life out and grow up. And it took hitting rock bottom for me to wake up. That's the moment I swam through the icy-cold pool and saw the light!

I am proud to say I was able to shift my life dramatically in under a year. I opened my first bank account (mind you, I needed a Xanax and had to hold the manager's hand while I did it!). Then I filed for bankruptcy and got rid of all the debt I was blissfully unaware that we had accumulated. I managed to gain more time before my house went into foreclosure, and I sold it by myself. At least the money I made from the sale paid for my bankruptcy attorney! With the help of my mom, dad, and stepmom, I cosigned on a lease and moved to an area that was best for my kids.

I got certified in Pilates and as a life coach. After the insane chaos I had gone through, and the 180-degree turnaround I made, I am beyond qualified to teach others how to change their lives for the better. Not only do I see solutions for people, in health, wellness, and life in general, but I can empathize as well. I've been in their shoes. I also expanded cLEAN Momma into a lifestyle brand for moms. My motto is "When life hands you lemons, make lemonade . . . then sell it on the corner and squat while you do it!"

DOWN AND DIRTY TIP: Whiter Whites, Brighter Brights

Throughout this book, I'll share some of my favorite cleaning tips in these Down and Dirty boxes.

Sometimes my whites turn gray and dingy. My girlfriend Melissa taught me this clever little trick: To brighten white linens, add ¼ cup lemon juice to the wash cycle.

You can also brighten colors by adding 1 cup vinegar to your wash.
Note: Don't use vinegar if you are using bleach—they're a dangerous combo!

A cLEAN Start

And now I have this book, a real opportunity to teach so many more tired, frazzled, fed-up, hardworking moms how to find themselves and make their lives easier. I learned that whining or bitching only keeps one stuck. Choices are for us to choose, and taking action helps you evolve and grow. The word *cLEAN* means much more than cleaning your countertops. It means cleaning out your *guts*, your life, your diet, your brain clutter. For me, what matters is the big picture: *life*. How do you live it, handle it? Are you present and aware? Can you solve problems? Do you face your issues or run from them? Do you appreciate what you have and own who you are? Do you follow your dreams, enjoy being loved and giving love in return? Are you able to let go of the past and move toward the future? Are you able to get off your butt and seize the life you were meant to live?

Don't mistake this for some cheesy self-help book. After having things handed to me for so long, then losing them all (and then some!), I have a unique outlook. I call it as I see it. My mom always told me, "Carolyn, the world is 4.5 billion years old! We are lucky if we make eighty-five years on this planet! How do you want to live your life? Embrace it. Go with it, enjoy it, own it, *live* it!" I finally got it, and I'm still working on it (and will probably *always* be working on it). But the point is, I am healthier and happier than I have ever been. I got my act together. My goal is to help you do the same—and I won't sugarcoat it. Most people need to scrub away a lot of crap in their lives and get their hands dirty. Are you ready to cLEAN up your act?

The cLEAN Momma Program

Okay . . . it all *sounds* good. But what will I have to do?

YOU'LL REDEFINE YOUR GOALS AND YOUR WAY OF THINKING. The cLEAN Mind-set is the clarity of goals and the belief that you can achieve anything you set your mind to.

YOU'LL CLEAN YOUR WAY TO A LEANER BODY. The cLEAN Momma Workout is a combination of cardio and strength-training exercises that allow you to multitask. Do you keep finding excuses not to exercise? This program is for you!

YOU'LL LEARN TO EAT HEALTHIER. The cLEAN Diet isn't about starving yourself to go to your high school reunion—it's about creating good long-term eating habits that you can live with. If you keep finding your hands in the potato chip bag without even realizing it . . . you've found your solution!

YOU'LL GET ORGANIZED AND IN CONTROL. The cLEAN Routine will show you how to simplify and de-clutter your home and your life.

YOU'LL HELP YOUR FAMILY LEAD HAPPIER, HEALTHIER LIVES. cLEAN Family is about encouraging your kids to embrace healthy foods and exercise and enjoy more quality time with Mom! When Momma is centered and a good choice maker, kids feel secure and can mirror this.

YOU'LL SEE YOUR BODY AND MIND CHANGE. This is not a crash program; it's about baby steps. You'll see results, but they won't be overnight. Researchers say it takes about thirty days to form a new habit, so you need to allow yourself time to adapt. If you want the new habit to stick, this is how to go about it—so commit.

YOU'LL LEARN TO STAY MOTIVATED. How many times have you started a diet or new exercise regime only to lose steam? cLEAN Momma will teach you how to stay on track.

cLEAN
Mind

1
The Tools You Need

cLEAN Momma Says... Be aware of how you self-sabotage. Take off the blinders; start getting unstuck!

YOUR CHAPTER 1 LAUNDRY LIST

A "laundry list" is simply a list of items or tasks that are important. You'll see one at the beginning of each chapter—it's my way of summing up what I want you to take away from reading. These lists will also bring you back to your focus: What's my goal? Why am I doing this? What do I need to get there?

- Arm yourself with the basic tools you need to cLEAN up your life.
- Understand that before your body can be healthy, your mind needs to be healthy as well.
- Open your eyes and your mind: be aware of what you do and why, and consider changing what's not working for you.
- Clear out the emotional obstacles that are standing in your way.

Just as every home needs the basic cleaning tools (a vacuum, a mop, a bottle of Windex, etc.), you need some tools to clean out your life. These are the things you can utilize when life gets messy and you need to restore balance and peace to your daily world. They will help you focus and forge ahead. They will help you appreciate what you have instead of gripe about what's missing. And they'll make it easier for you to get unstuck from the negative patterns that have been trapping you for so long.

I tried for years to assemble my toolbox. I bought about a million and one self-help books, and they just didn't speak to me or hold my interest (okay, maybe the ADD had a little to do with that!). I didn't want or need someone telling me I was screwed up and had to fix things. I already knew that, thank you. What I needed was to make some changes by myself, for myself. But I had no freakin' idea where or how to start.

Thanks to the journey I went through (my financial duress, my divorce, my near–nervous breakdown), I organically came to this awakening. Cheesy, I know, but unbelievably powerful and humbling. It was as though the seas parted! When you hit rock bottom, things suddenly become crystal-clear (although I wouldn't recommend it). I felt stripped down to my core, naked, *clean*. And, for once, I was able to see what really matters. I could put all the other things away—they were only cluttering my life more. If I drew upon these eight simple principles, the pieces all fell into place. I could follow the path without tripping over my own two feet.

Don't get me wrong. I still have days when I am not the epitome of grace under pressure (PMS sucks!). In fact, twenty minutes before writing this section, I lost it when I discovered my daughter and her BFF using all my spices to make soup in the bathtub! But the point is I've transformed my way of thinking. I've created this toolbox that I can dig into when I need to feel inspired and in control. Even when my bathroom stinks of paprika and cinnamon, I have the tools within me to draw upon.

Tool 1: Awareness

Being aware of something is not just seeing it. It's an opportunity to make a choice—a conscious decision to either move on or remain complacent and stuck. When life or circumstances get too overwhelming, it's really easy to shut down, to not take a good hard look at things. I used to be the queen of avoidance, until I realized how self-defeating and destructive that behavior was. When you have awareness, you can take action, good or bad, but at least you're accountable. You're in control of what you think, believe, do—no one else. It's empowering! Having awareness is imperative to leading an authentic life and moving forward with your goals.

- **BE AWARE OF WHAT YOU BELIEVE.** Your beliefs are what you act upon. So if you're walking around convinced you're "a worthless piece of crap," you're not going to ask for that promotion or move out of your parents' basement. But if you're aware of your beliefs, especially the negative ones—if you see that they're holding you back—you can put the wheels in motion to change.

- **BE AWARE THAT ANYONE CAN SCREW UP.** No one is 100 percent right all the time. Not you, not your husband, not your child's fifth-grade teacher. Just being aware of this can help you practice patience and forgiveness. For me, it keeps me from blowing my top when someone says something incredibly stupid or conceited. Let it go . . . We're all guilty of making stupid comments sometimes.

- **BE AWARE OF YOUR FEELINGS.** Let's say you've had a tough day, and you're unwinding in front of the TV, watching *Dancing with the Stars* while mindlessly munching on a bag of potato chips. So how does awareness fit in? Instead of shoveling junk food into your mouth, be aware of the emotion that is causing you to do this. Acknowledge, "I feel overwhelmed, tired, pissed off at the world!" Then, when you go for the bag of chips in your pantry, you'll be making a conscious choice to eat them: "I am eating these chips because I am entitled to them and I want to feel better in this moment." That's fine. Eat them. But at least hold yourself accountable. Having awareness doesn't necessarily stop you from eating the chips, but you're more likely to pour a few chips into a bowl rather than chow down on the entire bag.

- **BE AWARE OF HOW YOUR ACTIONS AFFECT OTHERS.** I'm not going to tell you how to behave—that's your business. I'm not your mommy. But I am going to ask you to be aware of how whatever you do can have a ripple effect on those around you. Let's just say you had a disagreement at work and now you're in a crappy mood. So you come home and you take it out on your kids or your husband. Were you aware that chewing them out would make them feel hurt/angry/sad? Or did you just act on your frustrations?

- **BE AWARE OF THE LITTLE THINGS.** Stop and smell the roses! Just being aware of the moment, of a pleasant fragrance, sound, taste, color, can elevate your mood. If you're tuned in to these tiny details, they add up. For me, it's taking in "the change" in nature: the way the leaves turn colors in the fall, how the flowers blossom in the spring. I love to stomp in puddles when it's raining and to make a cup of hot cocoa when it's cold outside.

- **BE AWARE THAT YOU ARE CHANGING.** Every second is an opportunity to grow and evolve. And when you seize that opportunity, give yourself some credit. Even baby steps are meaningful. When you do something positive to bring you closer to your goals, make a mental note of it.

Tool 2: Open-mindedness

If you haven't already figured this out, I am a person who likes to think outside the box. I don't like to feel confined to one way of doing something. My ideas can be a little wacky, but who gives a damn! When you're open-minded, nothing is impossible and no situation is hopeless. That said, it's not always easy to proclaim, "What the hell? I'll do it my way!" Maybe you were raised a certain way or you've been living with a situation for so long that doing anything different seems like a huge leap. I was raised to not take care of myself and to depend on other people—so that was normal for me. I needed to reboot. I'm not saying to compromise who you are or what you believe—just open the door (even a crack!) and let new ideas come in. There's a tremendous freedom in it— you'll never feel trapped again. The most successful people in the world are often the most flexible; the ones who go with the flow rather than resist change.

Tool 3: Moderation

Have you ever been totally excited and motivated to start a new diet? At first, you're into it, so you go balls to the wall, and you drop weight as fast as you use a roll of toilet paper.

Then, suddenly, you slow down. Your weight stays the same, and you get bored. You say to yourself, "I'm so in the mood for crispy French fries, I'll just have a few . . ." Soon you're on a slippery slope, and the next thing you know, it's "Hell, I'm getting a burger, some mac 'n' cheese, and a shake to go with my fries!" Soon after, you're back to your old, crappy habits, feeling bloated, five pounds heavier, and totally self-defeated.

Been there. Done that. About a bazillion times.

Then I figured out why moderation is the key. In order to stay motivated and continue moving forward, you have to tackle things with moderation. Bit by bit, corner by corner. I'm talking about making lifelong changes for yourself. Rome wasn't built in a day, girlfriend. When you make mini-goals for yourself and go at a slower pace, you have a higher likelihood of sustaining and plowing through the toughest obstacles. If you try to run a marathon before you can run around the block, I guarantee you will fall on your face!

Moderation also applies to the way you treat yourself. If you have been filling your face with sugar for ten years, you're not going to be able to go cold turkey the first week. Start slow; have one Oreo. It won't kill you. Craving a slice of pizza, have one . . . not the entire pie. Know when enough is enough. If you give in to a craving and have a candy bar, it doesn't mean that your diet is ruined and you should eat everything you want for the rest of the day. Finish your sweet, but make healthy food choices for the rest of the day. There's power in that control. And moderation is like a muscle. The more you flex it, the stronger it gets.

Tool 4: Motivation

Motivation means getting off your butt and *doing* something. Sometimes it's the hardest tool in my box. But I know that to succeed at anything, you must stay motivated. When you start something (a diet, an exercise program), your motivation is high. But two weeks later, it may start to fizzle. That's because we all want a quick fix. We want to see results *fast*. On top of that, your drive can constantly be under attack by your own negative thoughts and anxiety. It's hard to keep moving forward when something is holding you back. There are four big reasons that people lose motivation:

1. **YOU HAVE NO CONFIDENCE.** If you don't think you're going to succeed, then why the hell try?

2. **YOU LACK CLARITY.** You don't have a clue what you want or what's wrong.

3. **YOU HAVE NO DIRECTION.** If you don't set some goals, how will you reach them?

4. **YOU HAVE NO PATIENCE.** You start with a high level of motivation when you get into something new, then it peters out.

Luckily, all of the above are fixable. You can draw upon your other tools (awareness, moderation, gratitude) to help you plant the seeds and see the big picture. You have to outshout the negative voices in your head that are saying "Give up!" or "I can't!" You can. You will. Why? Because you're already taking the steps by reading this book. You're motivated to make some changes and rethink your game plan for your future. Ride that wave of positive momentum!

Here are some other great ways to get your motivation pumped:

- **GET OFF AUTOPILOT.** Stop doing the same things over and over again because you're used to them. Rock the boat just a tiny bit and you'll see how your motivation soars. It can be something very small, like setting your alarm clock for ten minutes earlier so you can squeeze in some stretching or meditation. Making just a small change can be the catalyst you need to keep going. Just reaching outside your comfort zone and taking risks is empowering.

- **ASK YOURSELF QUESTIONS THAT WILL HAVE POSITIVE ANSWERS.** What excites me? What makes me happy? What am I most proud of? Write the answers down and note how these things make you feel. This is a clue to the path you should be on. And it also helps you refocus on the good in your life instead of the bad.

- **FAKE IT TILL YOU MAKE IT.** If you don't feel particularly motivated, act as though you are. Smile, laugh, turn up the enthusiasm. In a few minutes, you may start to feel that way for real.

- **LET'S MAKE A DEAL.** You may not particularly feel like working out today, but tell yourself, "If I Taskercise and clean my kitchen for ten minutes, I'll sit down later with the kids and watch *American Idol*." It will help you over that hump of avoidance and procrastination if you know there's a little reward in store!

- **GIVE IT FIVE MINUTES.** Even if you're dreading doing something, commit to doing it for a very short period of time. That one little push can get you going.

- **PARTNER UP.** Sometimes having a friend to share with is a great motivator. He or she can give you a boost when you're feeling lazy or talk you down from a ledge when you want to quit.

- **CHOOSE TO BE HAPPY.** You don't *have* to be unhappy, unhealthy, and lost. No one is twisting your arm—that's your choice. If you want something more for yourself, then make the decision to do something about it. Plant the seed. You don't have to figure it all out yesterday, but when your brain opens up, ideas come flooding in at the weirdest times (like when you're having sex . . . just sayin'!). You may think your goal is impossible to achieve. Well, that's the difference between people who succeed and people who give up. They both have the same hurdles, but tenacity gives you the strength and courage to run toward the finish line.

- **GIVE YOURSELF A WAKE-UP CALL.** Every time your motivation starts to dwindle, remind yourself that you are worthy, capable, and committed. Better yet, set a smaller, attainable goal, and then rebuild. Beat it into your head! Which brings us to . . .

Tool 5: Decisiveness

Life is filled with indefinites—you can't always know the outcome of your actions before you make a move. But you can gather data and look at what it is you want to accomplish. The alternative is a hell of a lot worse—let's call it "limbo land." When you can't make a decision, you'll remain there, trapped forever in a place of ambivalence. And even if you do make a bad choice—you act out of fear or emotion (never a good idea!)—there is a lesson to be learned, regardless of the outcome. The more decisions you make, the better you'll get at evaluating situations and making choices based on information, not only your emotions. Action beats inaction any old day. Being decisive requires courage, wisdom, and confidence. The very act of making a choice will do wonders for your self-esteem.

Some things that might help you make up your mind:

- **GATHER YOUR INFO. Make an informed decision. If it helps you see things clearer, make a list of pros and cons. But . . .**

- **DON'T DRAG IT OUT FOREVER! This is called procrastinating, wavering, dragging your feet. Set a deadline and just do it; take the plunge!**

- **DON'T LET OTHERS SWAY YOU. Be your own person; make up your own mind.**

- **SURPRISE YOURSELF. Do something out of character, out of your comfort zone. It can be thrilling and exhilarating—just the kick in the butt you need.**

- **IMAGINE YOURSELF DOWN THE ROAD. How does this decision make you feel? Does it give you a sense of joy, peace, accomplishment? Then it's the right move to make.**

- **GO WITH YOUR GUT. Sometimes your instincts are the best barometer of whether or not the decision is the right one. Your gut speaks the truth; your brain justifies indecisiveness and keeps you vacillating.**

Tool 6: Calmness

What do you do when the rug is pulled out from under you? Do you lose your head/ mind, or do you remain calm? I know we've all been through tough times, but being able to stay calm in a crisis—either real or imagined—is an important tool. You don't have to be facing a firing squad to feel anxious; everyday situations and work/family emergencies do the trick just fine. They push you to the breaking point and you have to choose how you're going to handle it.

Calmness comes from balance. Calmness comes from security and from having a road map. Calmness comes from strength. Calmness comes from proper time management. I call upon this tool when I feel my blood pressure starting to rise over something out of my control. That's when I take a step back, look at the big picture, and try my damnedest not to blow things out of proportion. When we accept, and are calm about, our situations, people are more inclined to help us, and we are more inclined to solve problems. A few suggestions on how to keep your cool:

- **DON'T OVERDRAMATIZE. Ask yourself, "Does it matter?" Not everything that happens is a catastrophe, so you don't have to react as though it is. Seriously, we are too old to cry over spilled milk, scream at some dope who cut us off on the road, or get twirled up in a knot because some other mom at the playground is judging us. Life's too short!**

- **CHOOSE HOW YOU WILL RESPOND. You may be powerless to change the source of the stress, but you have the power to choose how you will react to it. Will you shake it off? Will you ignore it? Will you face it head-on without fear or intimidation? Be aware of the choices you can make, no matter how dicey the situation.**

- **BE AWARE OF YOUR TRIGGERS, the little things that set you off, make your blood boil. Just knowing you might be confronting a tense situation can help you keep your wits about you.**

- **TAKE IT ONE STEP AT A TIME. A big problem can feel overwhelming. Break it down into smaller pieces and focus on one small goal at a time.**

- **CREATE A CALM ENVIRONMENT. A place you can go to unwind—maybe it's your bathroom for a soothing bubble bath, or your bedroom where you can mellow out to music. Make your own "Momma Cave" to retreat to when you need to chill out.**

Tool 7: Confidence

Oh, yes, you can! Don't let fear and insecurity hold you back. Confidence truly is more that just walking around with a size 2 body with a million bucks in the bank and a shiny new Mercedes convertible. Confidence is actually competence. You're secure with yourself and feel efficient and capable in the world. This is inner strength and is so much more powerful than a closet full of couture!

When you are confident, you don't need to rely on superficial crap to make you feel good. Even in the toughest of times, when I didn't have a pot to piss in, I felt confident. Why? Because I was learning how to handle life's curveballs. I didn't give a damn that my best friend had more money and nicer shoes than I did. I was tackling something I had never done before—balancing my own checkbook! I rocked!

So how do you build your confidence?

- **DON'T LISTEN TO THAT NEGATIVE VOICE IN YOUR HEAD. The one that makes you uncomfortable, embarrassed, ashamed. Tell it to shut up! Maybe it's been there since you were a kid, but you're a grown-up now. You've moved past it. You're stronger and wiser.**

- **STOP FEELING SORRY FOR YOURSELF. Sometimes it's good to have a two-minute pity party and release the crap from your system. It's like shaking up a soda bottle and opening the top! It's healthier to release the emotion than stuff it down. But don't indulge and let it take over so you're wallowing in "woe is me" mode. Keep it to under five minutes, laugh at yourself, then focus on solution making and move forward.**

- **SMILE AT YOURSELF IN THE MIRROR. Researchers have a name for this: "facial feedback theory." It means that your expression can actually send a message to your brain. So say cheese! You might feel happier and more confident (or like a big dork!).**

Tool 8: Gratitude

Gratitude is an amazing tool that will transform your life, but more important, it is a way of life. How grateful are you? Do you appreciate how good you have it, or do you get caught up with bitching and complaining about what you don't have, your crappy day, or the idiot in line at the grocery store? Do you appreciate the people in your life—or do you hyper-focus on what they didn't do, and criticize?

One day not so long ago, when I barely had enough money for instant ramen noodles, my kids and their friends were all playing in the park. The friends' parents invited us to lunch, but I couldn't afford it. Instead of complaining, or even feeling

Four Ways to Show Gratitude

- **BE KIND TO STRANGERS.** Do something nice for someone you don't know. Give up your seat to an elderly person on the bus; compliment a woman's perfume in the elevator; say thank you when someone holds the door open for you. Random acts of kindness are great ways to work your gratitude muscle. It just feels good to do good!

- **GIVE SOMEONE YOUR FULL ATTENTION.** This has become much easier for me. It's a way to take the attention off of my own problems and focus on another person. It feels good to give. I make it a point to sit down and really listen to my kids and my friends. I look them in the eye; I respond with more than "Uh-huh." Just a few minutes of your undivided attention can make your little ones feel so happy and appreciated. The same goes for a partner, coworker, or spouse.

- **JUNK THE JEALOUSY.** Why should you resent someone for being successful or happy? Jealousy is your own fragile ego's cry for attention. It says, "Appreciate me! I'm just as good!" And you are. Self-worth comes from self-love. Use your other tools to help you readjust your views of yourself. Be aware of all the great things you have in your life; see the positives instead of dwelling on the negatives. Know that if you feel something is missing, it's in your power to obtain it.

- **SAY THANK YOU . . . AND MEAN IT.** When your husband does the dishes; when your boss lets you go home half an hour early; when your kids remember to throw their dirty clothes in the hamper. Appreciate the small gestures of respect and kindness that people make toward you. The more you show your gratitude, the more they'll do to earn it!

embarrassed, I took my kids home and made mac 'n' cheese. We ate it in a fort I made with chairs and blankets outside. I thought at that moment, *I am so grateful for this!* I had fresh air, trees, a tent made out of pink blankets, and my two delicious kids. I was the luckiest woman in the world.

Researchers say that people who practice gratitude are 25 percent happier. That's proof enough for me to count my blessings on a daily basis! Life is finite; nothing lasts forever. Which should make you all the more grateful for the things and people you have around you right now. Sometimes it takes a crisis—like losing a job, a marriage, a whole lot of money—to wake you up. When I practice gratitude, I feel so much more connected instead of isolated.

---

cLEAN Momma Pop Quiz: "Oops, I did it again!"

At the end of every chapter, you'll see these boxes. Don't think of it as a test! I simply pose these questions to help you bring out your awareness and find your motivation. These "quizzes" will help you to think, focus, act, and embrace the cLEAN life. They're also a mini–cheat sheet to applying the principles covered in each chapter.

As you've learned in this chapter, the key to the cLEAN lifestyle is to replace negative behaviors with positive ones. I love the KISS approach: Keep It Simple, Stupid. The best way for you to be aware of the negative behavior that is holding you back is to keep a little tally.

How many times a day do you . . .

_____ Say something negative about yourself in your mind or out loud—and, even worse, in front of your kids?

_____ Slouch, look down, avoid eye contact?

_____ Mindlessly eat off your kids' plates, munch when you're not hungry, nosh late at night or in front of the TV?

_____ Make excuses, avoid responsibility for your actions, act defensive, insist you're right?

_____ Procrastinate, allow things to pile up (until you're overwhelmed), avoid making decisions or choices?

Now, you're going to do the same for positive behavior.

How many times a day do you . . .

_____ Pat yourself on the back, pat your children on the back, compliment someone for a kindness or a job well done?

_____ Check things off your to-do list and feel a sense of accomplishment?

_____ Feel present and in the moment; don't feel distracted?

_____ Appreciate the little things?

_____ Do something nice for yourself—color your roots, polish your nails, take a bubble bath?

_____ Feel good about what you eat?

_____ Hold your head up high, make eye contact with the cashier at the supermarket, practice good posture?

In the first week or two, the negative tallies might outnumber the positive ones. That's okay; you're creating awareness and working toward new behaviors. The next step will be to catch yourself before you self-bash— and that will come, and the negative tallies will decrease. Take note of the changes you are making and give yourself some credit!

2
Strip Away Stress

cLEAN Momma Says... Stress will suck the air out of your lungs! Figure out what triggers your tension and you'll find ways to turn down the noise in your head, regroup, and reboot.

YOUR CHAPTER 2 LAUNDRY LIST

- Understand what stress is and how it gets in your way.
- Learn how to recognize the symptoms of stress.
- Practice ways to wipe out stress.
- Recognize your stress triggers before they drive you nuts.

Stress can get in the way—*big time*—of achieving a cLEAN life. It saps your energy; it keeps you frozen instead of moving forward. It makes you feel out of balance and out of whack! If you're like me, you're dealing daily with deadlines, demands, irritating people, places, and things that grate on your nerves. I wish I had a big magic eraser that could just wipe all my anxiety away—kind of like how I wipe my kids' crayon marks off the walls. But that's just not gonna happen. Stress is a part of life.

Maybe you know people who are stress junkies, who need the adrenaline rush to feel motivated. In small doses, stress does give you a kick in the pants. For example, when I knew I had a week left to finish this book, I panicked . . . then I sat down, focused, and wrote like a crazy woman. Stress was my friend! In an emergency, stress can save your life (e.g., when you slam on the brakes to avoid a collision, or jump out of the way when a bus is about to hit you). Some researchers even believe that short-term boosts of stress can strengthen the immune system and protect against some diseases, such as Alzheimer's.

But on a regular basis, stress is bad news. It can consume you. I remember when my marriage was strained, my kids were acting out, and I didn't have a cent in the bank, I literally felt like I was drowning. I was on the *Titanic* of stress! And it didn't just swallow me up, it manifested itself all over my body. I had killer migraines, back pain, and neck pain. I was popping ibuprofen like candy (which, in turn, gave me huge ulcers!). Even scarier, I was at a point where this tension felt *normal* to me. It had become a part of my life.

For those of you who have yet to experience this type of severe stress, I do not recommend it. When you're constantly living in panic mode, your mind and body pay the price. You feel overwhelmed and out of balance. Physically, you may become sick or plagued with aches and pains. In my case, I felt as though I was a self-destructive hamster on a wheel, yet I had no clue what I was running from or toward. Several panic attacks later, I decided it was time to take the reins and sort this all out. I needed to take some action. I needed to calm the hell down!

What Is Stress?

Stress is your body's normal physical response to situations that make you feel threatened or agitated. When you sense danger—whether it's real or imagined—the body's defenses kick into action, sounding an alarm ("Hey, Carolyn! WTF?!"). This reaction is stress, and it comes with a host of symptoms, everything from a racing heart and sweaty palms to dizziness, trouble breathing, and a rise in blood pressure. Your body is releasing a flood of hormones, including adrenaline and cortisol, and trying to get your attention!

Sometimes you may feel lousy, tired, cranky, out of sorts, and you don't know why. These are your body's not-so-subtle ways of signaling you that you're stressed out. Often, we chalk those symptoms up to other ailments or causes. I was convinced that my tension headaches were from a lack of caffeine, not from the fact that I had no idea how I was going to pay my bills and was going through a hellish divorce. Then I forced myself to admit it wasn't a lack of lattes; it was my own fear and frustration literally squeezing my head in a vice.

Stress feels differently to different people. For me, it's a pounding chest at three A.M., migraines, and forgetfulness. When I'm stressed, I always lose my car keys! A friend of mine tells me her stress sneaks up on her . . . like a dog that bites you out of the blue. She'll be walking down the street, perfectly fine, and suddenly she's overcome with anxiety. For a split second, she can't catch her breath. Some people feel frozen or paralyzed by stress. They literally can't move, react, or function. They may sleep more or retreat from normal activities. Others may feel anxious, breathless, and agitated—as if there's a gun being held to their head. Still others feel spacey or out of it, and may have trouble remembering or concentrating.

Stress can wreck your sleep, kill your appetite, or cause you to constantly eat. It can make you sad or pissed off at the world. It can leave you feeling lost and alone. When you're stressed, you are more likely to act out or make impulsive choices that are fear-based. You might beat yourself up or try to quell your nerves by eating junk or having a third glass of wine.

And its causes are equally varied: everything from relationship and money problems to work issues, life changes, or just plain burning the candle at both ends. I knew I was in deep doo-doo when I had all of the above going on in my life. I was a stress bomb ready to blow! But the last thing I wanted to do was analyze my situation. Hell no! I didn't want to look at my problems! It was too overwhelming. But once I took my

Is It Stress?

According to the American Institute of Stress (www.stress.org), there are dozens of common signs and symptoms of stress. Among them:

- Headaches
- Teeth grinding
- Stuttering
- Tremors/shaking
- Lightheadedness/dizziness
- Neck ache, backache, muscle spasms
- Ringing in the ears
- Rashes/itching
- Heartburn/gas
- Constipation or diarrhea

- Chest pain or palpitations
- Frequent urination
- Frequent sweating
- Lack of libido
- Anxiety/worry
- Insomnia
- Forgetfulness, trouble concentrating
- Anger
- Fatigue
- Weight gain or weight loss

thumb out of my mouth and uncoiled from the fetal position, I was able to see clearly what I needed to do.

cLEAN Solutions to Stress

It all boils down to two basic cLEAN Momma principles: awareness and action. Figure out what's freaking you out, then do something about it!

OPEN YOUR EYES. Identify what is going on in your life . . . really. You need to face the facts before you can wipe out the fear. Step outside your body and pretend to float up into the sky and look down into your world. What do you see? Once you've come clean with yourself, check in and see what you are doing to contribute to your own stress and anxiety. Are you adding fuel to the fire? Are you ignoring the elephant in the room? Instead of placing blame on others and on your circumstances, take a good look at what it is you do to contribute to this. What changes can you make? What ways can you reorganize your life to make things better, easier?

WRITE IT OUT. When you've identified the issue or issues plaguing you, it's time to take action. This means coming up with a road map. Take out a sheet of paper and write the word STRESSORS in the center of it. Now make a large circle around that word. Draw about half a dozen lines radiating outward from the circle, almost like a sun. Then write your stressors on each of the lines. For example, one line might say "kids," one might say "money," and another "work."

Circle the biggest stressor, then write down all the things about that stressor that are challenging you. For example, "Boss: criticizes, nags, blames, passed me over for promotion, demands long hours, unreasonable deadlines . . ." From there, take the priority, the most important stressor, and put that into the center of the circle, underneath STRESSORS. Then come up with your solutions.

The act of writing it out in this way helps your brain clearly see the path. There's something very soothing about putting your problems down on paper; it allows your brain to sift through the clutter and see things more clearly. What can you do to alleviate this stressor? In what ways can you be proactive? Things may not change overnight, but at least you have a plan. And that alone will decrease your anxiety and motivate you.

SLOW DOWN. I am guilty of constantly gunning the gas pedal. Sometimes my life feels as though it's on fast-forward and I can't slow down for a second—there's just too much to get done and too little time to do it in. Usually, it's my body that puts on the brakes. The last time I was speeding ahead, I came down with a lousy case of the flu. I was stuck in bed for days, completely debilitated. But I slept, I rested, I nourished, I recouped. And when I got back on my feet, I knew I had to be more realistic with my time and my tasks. It's okay to make lists and to check them off, but it's not okay to be in motion every second of the day. You need some down time. Give yourself a time-out if you feel your stress levels rising.

How to Breathe

Find a comfy place to either lie down or sit. Your back should be straight, your neck and shoulders relaxed. Let 'em drop.

Close your eyes and place one hand on your stomach, the other on your chest. Take a deep breath in through your nose, making your stomach expand like a balloon. Hold for a few seconds.

Slowly exhale through your mouth, pushing the breath out of your belly and into your lungs. Feel your tummy deflate. Do this ten or twelve times. As you breathe, your mind might wander and you may even get ants in your pants. So pick a word or two to repeat on your inhale and exhale. I like to say, "I am *calm*." You can say "strong," "grounded," "relaxed" . . . whatever word you connect with that soothes your fried nerves.

When you are finished, open your eyes and roll your head to the right then to the left.

BREATHE! Amazing how often we forget to do this simple act. Just open your mouth, take in some air, let it fill your lungs, and exhale. Ahhh . . . so much better! I am a big believer in deep, rhythmic breathing. Not only does it quiet the mind and relax the muscles, but it actually gets oxygen to the brain. Start small, one or two minutes in the morning and one or two minutes in the evening before bed. The key is to create a new habit for yourself. If you start in small increments, you're more likely to continue and feel successful at it. Then, once the habit is created, add an extra minute. Do this for ten minutes a day, *every* day. Even if you have to lock yourself in the closet, *do it!*

A PEACEFUL PICTURE. You're going to focus on a picture—it can be a painting on the wall or a photo on your computer screen, or something real, like a leaf on a tree just outside your window. Study the details, how the light reflects on it, the colors and shading, the shadows and texture. Don't allow any interruptions—no kids, phones, or e-mails should pull your attention away. Focus solely on sensing this image to the fullest; be in the moment. I find this process stills the noise in my head. It shifts the focus back to the present. Afterward, I'm calm, refreshed, and refocused.

SOUNDS OF SILENCE. Another way to quiet your screaming brain is to take five minutes and unplug. Turn off your music, TV, computer, phone, whatever is on. Sit or lie down for three to five minutes, simply tuning in to the world around you. Hear the car horns honking, the lawn mowers buzzing, the birds chirping. The goal is to be present and tap into the sounds around you, and let go of the noise in your head.

LAUGH. A good chuckle is good medicine for anxiety. I'll be honest . . . sometimes, when I feel like crawling out of my skin, breathing exercises just ain't gonna cut it. That's when I go for a giggle. Take a break and watch something funny. There's so much mindless crap that's hysterical on the Internet and TV. Or I'll call an old friend and reminisce about some random funny things we did. If all else fails, make yourself laugh. Look in the mirror and laugh out loud. Better yet, do it in your bra. You'll feel like the biggest dork and crack yourself up!

ACT LIKE A KID. Plop yourself down on the ground and hang with your kids. This is a win-win for everyone. You'll distract yourself from your worries and plug into your creativity, and they'll get uninterrupted Mommy and Me time. I find playing with Play-Doh the ultimate stress-buster. There is something about using my hands to shape, squeeze, and mold this mushy substance that takes me to a happy place. Maybe it reminds me of my childhood when my troubles were miles away? Whatever the reason, I am able to zone out and create with my kids. I wish I could carry those little cans of colorful clay in my purse and break 'em out whenever I need them!

CLEAN UP. I don't have to tell you that there is something seriously therapeutic about washing, wiping, and scrubbing the hell out of your home, do I? When I'm all in a lather, I lather up the dishes in my sink. I summerize or winterize my closet. I tidy up the kids' toy chest. I scrub my tiles with a toothbrush. When life is spinning out of control, these are things you *can* control. You can organize your home even if you can't clean up any of your other issues.

DOWN AND DIRTY TIP: Mildew Be Gone

Have you ever smelled your towels or clothes in the hamper and wondered what died in there?! There's a wet towel buried under the pile, and mildew has set in. No problem.

Try soaking the towel for ten to twenty minutes in distilled white vinegar diluted with water. The stinkier the mildew smell, the more vinegar (and less water) you'll need. Then, machine wash in hot water. Fresh as a daisy!

A SCENT-SATIONAL WAY TO CALM. I love to light a candle and watch the flame flicker and dance. The smell of the burning wax is intoxicating, especially if you choose a scent that's known for its aromatherapy properties. For centuries, people have used aromas to promote emotional and physical well-being. The amygdala, the brain's emotional center, is directly connected to the olfactory system. So when you smell a certain scent, it can trigger an emotional response. I like scented candles, but you can also pick up some essential oils or scented lotions and soaps.

DANCE IT OUT. Dancing around, alone or with your kids, is a great way to blow off steam—not to mention burn calories and power up your metabolism. You may feel

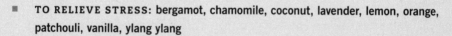

Scent-sations

- **TO RELIEVE STRESS:** bergamot, chamomile, coconut, lavender, lemon, orange, patchouli, vanilla, ylang ylang

- **TO REDUCE ANXIETY/FEAR:** bergamot, chamomile, cedarwood, frankincense, jasmine, lavender, mandarin, neroli, patchouli, rose, sandalwood

- **TO EASE DEPRESSION/FATIGUE:** basil, clary sage, frankincense, ginger, grapefruit, jasmine, lemon, orange, rose, rosemary, peppermint, sandalwood, vanilla, ylang ylang

like a dork (especially if you're like me, and you dance with your kids on the coffee tables!), but you'll be a dork in a good mood! Allow yourself to feel the music, move your arms, and sway your body, letting the tension drain. This puts you in the moment for sure!

CHILL OUT! Incorporate a cold shower into your routine. It gives you an instant rush, leaving you feeling refreshed and revitalized. For me, it's like hitting "reboot" when I'm stressed. Cold water releases natural endorphins into your bloodstream and brain. It shifts your mood. There are many scientists who even believe cold showers can help alleviate symptoms of depression. If you can't take the cold water off the bat, it's okay to start warm and gradually decrease the temperature. Stand under a cold shower for as long as you can. Relax into it. This shocks the nervous system and helps rewire the brain. I like to switch numerous times between hot and cold water, and end the shower with cold water.

cLEAN Momma Pop Quiz: What Stresses You Out?

Ask ten different people what stresses them out, and you're likely to get ten different answers. Stress is very personal, and not everyone is affected by it in the same way. What freaks someone out may not faze you, and vice versa. So you can get a grip on what flips you out, write the numbers 1–12 next to these top stressors (1 being the least; 12 being the most). Look at your list—what can you control? What can you do to alleviate the stress you feel surrounding this issue? The idea is to understand your stress triggers better, so tension doesn't taint all the good stuff in your life. Consider how you are going to handle your major stressors, numbers 8–12. Focus on concrete, realistic steps.

_____ Major life changes (new baby, new home, divorce, death, etc.)

_____ Money

_____ Spouse/partner

_____ Kids

_____ Friends/neighbors/acquaintances

_____ Work

_____ Health

_____ Family (parents, siblings, in-laws)

_____ Weight

_____ World problems (e.g., politics, poverty, pollution)

_____ Your schedule/deadlines

_____ Growing older

3
Polish Up Your Ego

cLEAN Momma Says . . . Stop being a doormat, comparing yourself to others, and complaining about what's wrong with you. Focus on what's right!

YOUR CHAPTER 3 LAUNDRY LIST

- Devote some time to yourself: your needs, your desires, your feelings, your body.
- Notice if you are being your own worst critic—and silence the negativity.
- Realize that no one is perfect . . . and you don't have to be.

Motherhood can give you amnesia. It makes you entirely forget who you are. You focus on being "Momma" and all of a sudden forget you're also a person. Life becomes all about your kids, and your needs, wants, desires, and dreams . . . well, you might as well chuck 'em in the Diaper Genie.

But hear me out: when you stop caring about yourself, everything else pays a price. You feel less desirable, less sexy, less confident, and unworthy. Then you get angry and frustrated and beat yourself up. When you enter this place, you are more likely to eat crap, gain weight, stop exercising (or never start), and basically give up on yourself. Welcome to the world of low self-esteem!

I am very familiar with this feeling, because I lived with it most of my life. Even in college, I was insecure. I compared myself to my friends. I never felt competent. So how did my self-loathing turn to self-respect? I stopped trying to force people, things, or circumstances to change and accepted things for what they were. I realized I had choices and I could make choices. I learned that getting validation from outside sources only made me feel good for the moment. In order for me to truly feel good about myself, I needed to rely on me! I put together a plan to boost my ego and pull myself out of the shadows and into the spotlight.

RETRAIN YOUR BRAIN. Pay attention to how often you say self-destructive things about yourself. How many times a day do you announce, "I'm fat! My butt looks huge in these jeans!" or "I'm so lame! I can't . . ." Also take note of how often you say these things out loud and in front of your kids. Do you think it's a good idea for your children to hear their mommy say negative things about herself? Most likely, they will grow up mirroring this behavior and feeling negatively about their own self-worth. So stop it!

Rule of thumb: If you don't have something nice to say about yourself, keep your mouth shut! Go back to your toolbox and dig out your awareness. Catch yourself thinking icky thoughts or saying icky words. You know, that nagging little voice inside your head that says "You suck" or "You look like crap." Over time, listening to a negative inner voice will torpedo your self-esteem. Replace your negative thoughts or words with ones that are proactive and positive. That doesn't mean you should go around singing, "I'm too sexy!" It simply means instead of telling yourself "I feel so fat," replace that sentence with "I'm so proud of myself, I ate really well this morning!" Be kind to yourself.

RESPECT YOURSELF. When you do, others will respect you. When you practice self-respect, you stand up for yourself, put yourself first, and do things for others not because you need to (or feel guilty and obligated to) but because you want to. It means holding true to your values and principles before anyone or anything else. It's trust-

If you can't say something nice . . .

Then write it down! I want you to jot down three positive things you can say to yourself to replace the negative mind chatter. Stumped for things to say? How about "I am a great mother to my kids"; "I am a great cook"; "I have beautiful blue eyes"; "I broke a million on Temple Run!" You get the picture.

1.

2.

3.

ing that if you are feeling a certain way, there is a legitimate reason behind it, and not second-guessing or apologizing for it.

APPLAUD YOUR VICTORIES . . . EVEN THE SMALL ONES. You grouted your tub; you got the kids off to school on time; you didn't forget your big bro's birthday. Congrats . . . you deserve a medal! Or at least a pat on the back. Don't belittle yourself all the time. Give some credit where credit is due. In your busy, hectic, harried life, being punctual, persistent, and tidy are all reasons to revel in your wonderfulness. I just took a shower and conditioned my hair . . . yay, me! Be aware when you get things done and get things right, and celebrate.

DO SOMETHING YOU ARE GOOD AT. Jump into a new passion or revisit an old hobby. Whatever makes you feel accomplished, competent, or talented, just do it! Trying something new is also a huge confidence boost. It shows you're a risk taker, and you have the courage to push your limits. Maybe there's something you've *always* wanted to do—like salsa dancing, or stained-glass sculpting, or gourmet cooking. What are you waiting for? Doing something artistic and expressive is particularly empowering; it lets you get those creative juices flowing and gives you an outlet for releasing any feelings trapped below the surface.

PUT YOUR BEST FACE FORWARD. Comb your hair; don't wear clothes that are stained or wrinkled; take the time to touch up your roots; fix a chipped mani. I understand: sometimes putting on yesterday's sweatpants crumpled up on the floor by the side of your bed is easier to do than finding something cute and fresh to wear. But this behavior can become a slippery slope! The next thing you know, your hair is greasier than last night's dishpan left in the sink, and your legs are a cross between Cousin Itt and Chewbacca. Try not to get stuck in this "Who cares about me?" rut. I care; you should care. Trust me, your significant other cares. Your outward appearance is often a projection of your inward self. Show the world you're worthy!

STAND UP TALL. The way you carry yourself can boost your self-esteem. Are you hunched over? Dragging your feet? Or are your shoulders back and your head held high? Are you making eye contact and smiling warmly . . . or nervously fidgeting? So much of our communication is done through body language. Your body language can have an effect on how other people perceive you, but it can also have an effect on how you perceive yourself. When you're walking anywhere, it feels natural to lower your head slightly and watch your step, but try to keep your chin up and eyes forward.

TREAT YOURSELF BETTER: Even Cinderella got a day off for good behavior! You are entitled to some R&R and pampering. You have my permission to spoil yourself—it will do wonders for your self-worth. Even if you don't have a ton of time, you can find fifteen minutes to:

- **Toss out your ratty granny panties and order some sexy new undies online.**

- **Deep-condition your hair.**

- **Make a cup of tea and catch up on your fave soap.**

- **Reconnect with old friends on Facebook.**

- **Dim the lights, play your fave sexy song, pour yourself a glass of wine, and chill!**

- Polish your toes, defuzz your legs, or loofah yourself in the shower.

- Soak in a warm, fragrant bubble bath.

- Slather on a face mask.

- Browse on eBay and treat yourself to a trinket.

- Bury your head under the blankets and just close your eyes!

SPEAK UP. Don't be afraid to give your opinion, to raise your hand, to make your voice heard. Don't start out with an intimidating situation (like a big brainstorming meeting with the boss). Instead, find a friendly group and say just one thing at every meeting. A friend of mine joined a book club so she could practice asserting her opinions. She wound up theorizing about *The Hunger Games* for a half hour in front of six fellow readers. Mission accomplished!

SURROUND YOURSELF WITH POSITIVITY. Hang out with people who care about and appreciate you. If your friends and family are constantly giving you unwarranted criticism, this can lead to low self-esteem. Have a talk with the people in your life about how negatively their harsh comments affect you; if they truly care for you, they'll put a stop to it immediately.

SET SOME BOUNDARIES. It's okay to say no! As moms, we tend to be people

DOWN AND DIRTY TIP: Fluff Stuff

If your child's favorite teddy is filthy, pour a capful of baby shampoo into warm water. Dampen a washcloth with the soapy mix and gently rub the stained areas in circles. Rinse with a clean, damp cloth and let air-dry. For super-duper dirt on a plush pal, check the label: you may be able to put it in the washing machine. Place it in a pillowcase, knot so Teddy stays tucked inside, then wash in Woolite on a gentle setting and tumble dry on low.

pleasers, sacrificing what's good for us in order to make other people happy. But all this mommy martyrdom causes resentment and stress. Don't be a doormat. If a task is too much for you to handle, avoid making up some lame excuse. Stand up for yourself and say, "No. I can't." This may be a challenge at first, but it will empower you! Don't tackle too many projects at once. Focus on a few that you really can channel your energy into. If you overcommit, it takes the fun out of the experience, and you'll just wind up resenting it!

Failure Is Not an F-Word!

Realize that failure or being wrong will not kill you. The world won't come to an end if you screw up. You learn from every mistake, growing as a person and becoming stronger, wiser, more experienced, and capable. I was at the final callbacks for Maureen, one of the leads in the Broadway national tour of *Rent,* and I decided I could just rehearse once or twice and learn the lyrics. Hell, I'd just wing it. Humungo mistake. I came off like an idiot. I was too young, too green, too overconfident. I was a disaster. Lesson learned: when an opportunity presents itself, put 200 percent into it. Be prepared like a freakin' Girl Scout. If you fall on your face when you gave it your best shot, at least you gave it your best shot. You can walk away, head held high. It was a wake-up call for me that you can't coast through life. Everything worth having takes effort. And the next audition . . . I got cast!

---

cLEAN Momma Pop Quiz: Does Your Self-Esteem Suck . . . or Soar?

Answer TRUE or FALSE to the following statements, then check your score below. And be honest with yourself!

_____ I excel at my work.

_____ I am happy.

_____ I am proud of myself.

_____ I can accept criticism.

_____ I am worthy of love.

_____ I am attractive.

_____ I don't need others' approval.

_____ People like me.

_____ I deserve respect.

_____ I am a good person.

If you answered 8–10 TRUE, then you've got a healthy ego!

If you answered 4–7 TRUE, you could use a little boost in the confidence department. Make sure to do the tasks in this chapter.

If you answered less than 4 TRUE, your self-esteem needs an extreme makeover. Try repeating each of the above statements to yourself every day and meaning it!

cLEAN
Diet

4

Eating cLEAN

cLEAN Momma Says ... cLEAN eating is not a quick fix; you won't lose a ton of weight overnight. But you will keep it off!

YOUR CHAPTER 4 LAUNDRY LIST

- Observe what you eat, how often, and why.

- Start by making small changes in your eating: Take it one step at a time. No drastic, crash dieting.

- Understand what cLEAN eating is all about—the types of food that will help your body look and feel better and give you more energy, strength, and stamina.

I hate the word *diet*. It makes me want to rebel and cheat, hide in my room, lock the door, and bust out a bag of Oreo cookies. I have been on many of the typical diet plans . . . and while they may work great for a bunch of folks out there, they didn't for me. Why? Because they involved short-term thinking. After my second child was born—and no pants would pull up past my thighs!—I came to the realization that it was time to think long-term, big-picture. I also had to get at the "why?"

First off, I was mindlessly eating processed crap. The playground? Nibble the kids' goldfish crackers. Watching TV at night? Rummage through the fridge and eat a whole second dinner while watching *So You Think You Can Dance*. I would take a heaping spoonful of peanut butter, ram it into a bag of chocolate chips, and shove it in my mouth, continuing till I felt physically ill.

Over the years, my longtime friend and registered dietitian Stephanie Lecovin and her hubby, Geoff, (www.nutritionhousecalls.com) witnessed many of my bad habits and kindly staged an intervention. I took it with a grain of salt, until I realized that she might be worth listening to. It was hard to admit to myself that I needed to create new habits. But what she said made sense, and the proof was in my ever-expanding butt: I needed to change. I needed to look at food differently. Once I dialed into a new mind-set, I began to view my choices differently. It took me some time, but eventually I began to see it in the way that Stephanie put it: "Eat real food and be aware that you're eating it."

When I expressed how I could never live without pizza, chocolate, or chips, she replied, "Then have pizza, but make it good pizza and sit down to enjoy it! Have chocolate, but make it good-quality dark chocolate. There are tons of healthier chips out there. Make sure you can recognize all of the ingredients in them as food, and be conscious when you eat them."

I thought about this and finally came to the conclusion that not only is she right, but this is very doable! The changes we're talking about here are meant to last for the rest of your life. Because this is a lifestyle change, you're going to gradually ease into it. Don't pressure yourself into going cold turkey. If you put a lot of pressure on yourself and make your diet radically different and restrictive right away, you'll cheat, feel guilty, and wind up comforting yourself with food. It's a vicious cycle!

I suggest you take your time and set out to learn bit by bit, creating new eating habits along the way. Don't do it to lose weight. Do it to be healthy and happy. Trust me, the weight will come off naturally and stay off.

Getting Started

Here are a few things I did in the first week that had an impact on me (and my body). The first steps are about getting your head in the game.

- **KEEP A FOOD JOURNAL.** This is about being present and conscious of your food choices. This was so key for me. I paid attention to my food intake and kept a journal for a month. I was so totally clueless about what I was eating until I saw it in black and white in front of me. That's a smack of reality for you! By doing this, I was able to see how inconsistent I was with my food intake. One day I would stuff my face, while another day I would basically deplete my body of energy by not eating enough.

- **EAT A VARIETY OF FOODS.** This is coming from the girl who grew up eating a peanut butter and jelly sandwich every day for lunch! You need to change it up a bit. Making your meals more interesting prevents boredom . . . and snacking later on. If you *always* have a bagel and cream cheese for breakfast, then try egg whites, cereal, yogurt, and fruit. Wake up those taste buds! You have so many more options out there. I look at it as a great opportunity to experiment with recipes and roam the aisles of my grocery store. Make sure your meals are chock-full of proteins, greens, and colorful fruits. I love a pretty plate with a rainbow of foods on it!

- **EAT SMALLER PORTIONS.** Just because my mother's meatballs and spaghetti is by far the best-tasting meal on this planet, I don't need to eat three pounds of it. That's what leftovers are for! As a visual guide, you should not eat a portion that is larger than the size of your fist. If you've got big hands, you've lucked out. Banish *seconds* from your vocabulary, and eat off of smaller plates. This helps trick your mind into thinking your portions are larger than they are.

- **DRINK MORE WATER.** I hated H_2O. I just couldn't bring myself to drink it. Let's be honest . . . it's tasteless. Diet soda was my poison of choice for years, until I learned that the aspartame in diet soda breaks down into formaldehyde in the body. You might as well drink out of the jar in chemistry class (be sure to remove the dead frog first!). Water keeps you hydrated while flushing out toxins. I suggest adding lemon juice and

How to Sneak Water into Your Day

Water is not exactly the tastiest beverage . . . in fact, it has no taste at all! For some people, this is a turnoff. But you can make it much more desirable and increase your daily intake, if you . . .

- **ADD FRESH FRUIT**, such as lemon, lime, or orange slices. You can even crush fresh berries or watermelon in your glass to tickle your taste buds.

- **FRESHEN IT UP** with cucumber or mint—especially in summer, it's a cool twist.

- **ADD A SPLASH OF JUICE**, something a little tart like cranberry, grape, or pomegranate—delish! Juices also contain vitamins and antioxidants (an added plus).

- **TRY IT BUBBLY.** Some people prefer sparkling to flat water. Mineral water or seltzer, or even no-cal flavored seltzers, are all good options.

- **SIP TEA.** There are tons of herbal and caffeine-free varieties that are healthy, fragrant, and refreshing, either hot or iced.

ice and tricking yourself into thinking you're drinking lemonade. I actually like it now . . . but more important, I like the way my body feels when it's not parched like the Sahara Desert.

- **EAT FREQUENT, SMALL MEALS.** This way, you won't feel utterly depleted when mealtime rolls around. Animals graze, and we're animals. You should be eating every two to three hours. Bottom line: if you're famished, you'll binge. When I started incorporating healthy snacks into my routine, it stopped me from pigging out later on. I discovered that snacking before I crashed enabled me to make healthier choices rather than reach for the quick fix (e.g., a Big Mac!).

- **PUT SMART SNACKS WHERE YOU CAN FIND THEM.** Stephanie encouraged me to keep handy little snack bags of high-powered foods (see the list on page 49). I now store them in my purse, my car, the front of my fridge. If it's in front of my face, I will eat it.

Smart Snacks

Here's what I reach for when I need a pick-me-up. Each of these satisfies my cravings for sweet, salty, or crunchy.

- A small apple or pear cut up with 1 Tbsp. peanut butter

- A handful of raw almonds or pecans, with ¼ cup berries

- A string cheese, or a small piece of low-fat cheese, with seven or eight pita chips, soy chips, pretzels

- Three hard-boiled eggs without the yolks

- Half an avocado drizzled with balsamic vinegar and a dash of salt and pepper

- Half a small tortilla stuffed with 3–4 Tbsp. chunky salsa (you can add a ton of veggies to make a veggie wrap)

- A fresh fruit cup and 1 Tbsp. low-fat yogurt

- A large artichoke (they're not just for dinner). Steam it for 45 minutes until it's soft inside and the leaves come off easily. Then, make a dipping sauce from lemon juice, salt and pepper, 1 tsp. each olive oil and balsamic vinegar, and heat it up in the microwave for 15 seconds.

- Baked broccoli. Get out a cookie sheet and cut up broccoli into small pieces. Drizzle with olive oil and lemon juice, and sprinkle with salt and pepper. Bake on high heat (400°F) for 30 minutes, till it gets crunchy. It's like eating a bag of greasy potato chips, but it's broccoli. Win-win!

So I did all of this for a month, gently reprogramming my body and my brain. And then guess what happened? I became a different person. My energy soared. I felt more satisfied and less irritable. I learned how to make smart choices with food, and I began to teach my kids the importance of eating well. It was a freakin' miracle. I was then ready to start the cLEAN Diet and to really embrace a healthy lifestyle, one meal at a time.

cLEAN Diet 101

First of all, you need to know there's more than one right way to eat. We all have different bodies, different metabolisms and genetics, and very different food preferences. You'll find what works for you, but there are a few general principles that Stephanie taught me that apply to everyone embarking on this program.

EAT FOOD. I know this might sound ridiculous, but let's face it, most Americans are filling their bodies with food products that are made to resemble food but are far from the real deal. If a food does not have a label, it is most likely real food (an apple or yam, for example). If a food does have a label, and either (a) you can't picture the ingredients growing, (b) you can't pronounce those ingredients, or (c) it takes you a good part of the day to read those ingredients, then in all likelihood, that product is not based on whole foods. Pick up a can of diet soda and read the label . . . see what I mean? Avoid all artificial colors and all artificial sweeteners.

FOCUS ON PROTEIN-RICH FOODS of the highest quality you can afford (sustainable fish, grass-fed meat, hormone- and antibiotic-free poultry, wild game); nuts and seeds; seasonal fruit and colorful veggies (organic, whenever possible); tons of greens. Keep starches (including starchy veggies like potatoes) and sugars to a minimum.

ENJOY YOUR FOOD. If you're going to eat ice cream, eat the real deal and enjoy it! You can't truly enjoy eating if you're ridden with guilt, so knock it off. You also can't

These Ingredients Are No-nos!

Here are some of the ingredients to avoid if you're reading labels. If you see these words, read no further. Just don't eat it!

- **HIGH-FRUCTOSE CORN SYRUP.** It's not that a small amount of this is so bad for you; it's that it's found in so many food products, very few of which are actually healthy.

- **PARTIALLY HYDROGENATED OILS (ALSO CALLED "TRANS FAT").** Without a doubt, this is the most harmful kind of fat you can eat. It's used by food manufacturers to add a creamy texture to baked goods (or for deep frying) and to extend shelf life, all the while contributing to heart disease and obesity. Pass!

- **ARTIFICIAL DYES (E.G., RED 3, YELLOW 6, BLUE 2).** These dyes are linked to cancer. Seeing them on an ingredient label is a clue that the food product is unhealthy.

- **PRESERVATIVES, SUCH AS SODIUM NITRITE.** Also linked to cancer, especially in children and pregnant women. Find nitrite-free hot dogs and lunch meats whenever possible.

truly enjoy eating if you're distracted, so turn off the TV or turn away from your computer and enjoy the food you're putting in your mouth.

IDENTIFY POTENTIAL FOOD ALLERGIES/SENSITIVITIES. We can be sensitive or allergic to some of the foods we eat. This can slow down metabolism as well as cause water retention. If your body feels funky (e.g., bloated, gaseous, queasy) after you eat something, jot it down. Your body is trying to tell you something! A lot of people have unidentified issues with gluten. Taking gluten-containing grains out of your diet can help tremendously with weight loss if you have a sensitivity. Even if you don't, taking out gluten can help by cutting many of foods that tend to pack on the pounds, including pastas, breads, cookies, pastries, muffins, bagels, and crackers.

EAT SMALL, FREQUENT MEALS. Eating every two hours helps keep blood-sugar levels stable. Unstable blood sugar can affect insulin sensitivity, resulting in fat storage. Dips in your blood sugar can also churn up cravings! Strive to eat five or six times a day. Here's a sample schedule:

> **BREAKFAST: 7:00 A.M.**
> **SNACK: 10:00 A.M.**
> **LUNCH: 12:30 P.M.**
> **SNACK: 3:00 P.M.**
> **DINNER: 6:00 P.M.**
> **OPTIONAL SNACK: 8:00 P.M.**

GO PRIMAL. Eating mostly vegetables, with some fruit, nuts, and a little meat (red, poultry, pork, fish) is a healthy way to boost your metabolism and keep insulin levels stable.

DRINK YOURSELF HEALTHY. Stay away from sweetened drinks and juices (even all-natural juices, except fresh vegetable-based juice). They raise your blood sugar very quickly and cause insulin to spike, leading to fat storage. Drink plenty of water. If you need additional hydration (from exercise or intense heat), drink diluted (50/50) coconut water. Avoiding alcohol will further help you to drop weight if you currently drink. If you want to drink alcohol, a glass of red wine is the best option.

CHART: cLEAN Momma Food Journal

I tell my clients to keep a log next to their kitchen sink, along with a pen. Never move this log. (Outta sight, outta mind!) Most moms are always at the kitchen sink, so you will see it there . . . and use it.

	WHAT I ATE/DRANK	I ATE AT HOME/OUT	I WAS FULL/HUNGRY AFTER	MY MOOD WAS . . .	MY ENERGY WAS (HIGH/LOW/MEDIUM)
DAY TIME					
DAY TIME					
DAY TIME					
DAY TIME					
DAY TIME					
DAY TIME					
DAY TIME					

The cLEAN Momma Healthy Plate

- **ONE QUARTER PLATE:** choose a protein (preferably organic and without hormones or antibiotics)—fish, chicken or turkey without skin and fat, grass-fed meat, shellfish, beans or lentils, tempeh or tofu

- **ONE QUARTER PLATE:** choose a starch (yams, sweet potatoes, squash, peas, corn, quinoa, brown rice, etc.)

- **ONE QUARTER PLATE OR MORE:** choose a variety of nonstarchy veggies, including (but not limited to):

  Asparagus

  Artichokes

  Beets

  Broccoli

  Brussels sprouts

  Cabbage

  Carrots

  Cauliflower

  Celery

  Dark, leafy greens (chard, romaine, spinach, arugula, kale, collards, etc.)

  Fennel

  Green beans

  Mushrooms

  Onions

  Peppers

The cLEAN Eating Plan Lite

If you've been living solely on ice cream, Big Macs, and Doritos, you can't just give it up tomorrow and start eating quinoa. Well, you can . . . but I don't recommend it. This approach can only lead to disappointment. Eventually, you'll feel deprived, start craving your old favorites, and fall back into bad habits. Allow your body and mind to adjust to this new nutritional way of thinking. When you are ready, you can dive into the next chapter with confidence! You'll embrace the cLEAN eating plan, as I did. I now have a palate for whole, organic foods and not processed junk. I can taste the difference and feel the difference in my body. But I needed to reach that point. Stephanie encouraged me to open my eyes to dark chocolate (who knew it was just as tasty as a Snickers?) and eat whole-grain bread instead of white. This plan is a philosophy for eating; the cLEAN and simple approach. Food should be as close to its original state as possible, not filled with preservatives, dyes, and god knows what else.

But let's not forget, you're a busy momma. You need convenience. You need to grab and go. You need to cook a meal in ten minutes while you're doing a load of laundry. I get it. So here's the "Lite" version of the plan to get you started. Take it one step at a time, and realize that to be successful, you have to want to change. You can't have the "so what" attitude about your eating all the time. You have to evolve, even if it's slowly. You may want to stay on this plan for a few weeks until you get used to it. You'll find that you will lose weight—as much as two pounds a week. Then, when you start the more intense thirty-day cLEAN Eating Plan (in chapter 5), your body will be prepared and you'll be less likely to go from one extreme to another and cheat. You'll stick to it, you'll have a higher level of motivation, and you'll be doing it for a different reason: not just to be thin but to be healthy as well.

Seven Days of cLEAN Eating: The Right Lite Plan to Get You Started

Use this as a guide for your first week. If you don't like high-fiber cereal, then don't eat it. If quinoa makes you gag, go for something else. It's important to eat what you like instead of force-feeding yourself. Any time a client of mine has followed a strict diet with food that tastes like crap, she's eventually thrown in the towel. I encourage you to eat foods you enjoy . . . still keeping things sane and healthy. If there's a comfort food you have to have, I say, eat it! But just a little bit, and savor it. A word to the wise . . . If you deprive yourself, you'll end up bingeing on potato chips at eleven thirty P.M., watching reruns of *Sex and the City* (not that I've ever done that . . .).

BREAKFAST

- Two multigrain waffles topped with 2 Tbsp. low-fat yogurt and ¼ cup blueberries or raspberries. Blueberries are higher in antioxidants and lower in sugar, but you can mix it up.

- ½ cup high-fiber cereal (I like Kashi Go Lean) and skim milk. Make sure the cereal has more than five grams of fiber per serving; you can also add ¼ cup berries for more.

- ½ cup high-fiber oatmeal with ¼ cup blueberries or raspberries. I like to chop up a small apple and eat it in my oatmeal with a handful of raw almonds. It adds a great crunch and a little sweetness (not to mention more fiber and protein).

- Two-egg-white omelet with ¼ cup shredded low-fat mozzarella cheese and assorted veggies (I mix in chopped spinach, mushrooms, bell peppers, and onions). You can eat this with a slice of whole-grain, high-fiber toast.

- Fruit smoothie. Blend ¼ cup berries with ¼ cup ice.

- Rush-and-go breakfast. On days when I'm crazed, I reach for a low-fat yogurt and a small handful of raw almonds, or a high-fiber, low-sugar breakfast bar such as Kashi Go Lean or Luna brand.

LUNCHES

- One four-to-six-ounce chicken breast. I bake mine in the oven at 400°F for 25–30 minutes, with a little garlic and lemon juice, plus salt and pepper. Chop it up and eat over a salad, on a whole-grain pita or slices of bread, or with a side of veggies. So versatile, so tasty.

- Simple salad. Opt for leafy greens (such as mesclun, spinach, kale) instead of romaine or iceberg (darker greens generally have more nutrients). Top with some protein, such as ½ cup chopped chicken breast, three hard-boiled egg whites, ½ cup low-fat cottage cheese, ¼ cup shredded low-fat mozzarella cheese, canned light tuna, lentils, or black

cLEAN Momma's Famous Dressing

This stuff is the bomb! I mix it up and keep it in my fridge to use as a dipping sauce, salad dressing, or a spread on my pita pockets and wraps.

MAKES 2 SERVINGS

3 Tbsp. fresh lemon juice

¼ cup balsamic vinegar

½ tsp. salt

¼ tsp. fresh ground pepper

2 Tbsp. light ranch dressing

2 Tbsp. grated Parmesan cheese

2 Tbsp. extra virgin olive oil

Combine the lemon juice, vinegar, salt, pepper, ranch dressing, and cheese in a medium bowl. Whisking constantly, add the oil in a thin stream.

You can store this dressing covered in the fridge for up to a week.

beans. Other salad toppers I love: ¼ cup raisins, 2 Tbsp. dried cranberries, ¼ cup crushed raw almonds, ½ cup salsa.

- ¼ cup grains (brown rice, whole-grain pasta, bulgur wheat, quinoa) topped with veggies (bell peppers, mushrooms, artichoke hearts, beets, carrots, cucumbers, tomatoes, radishes).

- High-fiber pita or tortilla stuffed with ¼ cup hummus and arugula, spinach, tomatoes, cucumbers, or veggies of your choice.

- High-fiber pita or tortilla filled with chicken breast or turkey slices, ¼ cup shredded low-fat mozzarella, veggies, and mustard (or cLEAN Momma's Famous Dressing).

- High-fiber tortilla wrap stuffed with 1 Tbsp. peanut butter and fresh berries. Heat in the microwave for 30 seconds.

- Turkey, chicken, or vegetarian chili topped with ¼ cup shredded low-fat mozzarella cheese, ¼ cup chopped tomato, ¼ cup diced onion, and 1 Tbsp. low-fat sour cream.

DINNER

- Chicken Marsala. I season eight or ten boneless, skinless chicken tenderloins with garlic powder, salt, and pepper. Then I lightly flour both sides and cook them in a covered skillet with four cut-up shallots, pre-sliced mushrooms, ½ cup Marsala wine, and ¼ cup chicken stock. Cook for 2–3 minutes over high heat; then let simmer over medium-low heat for 12–15 minutes, stirring or flipping occasionally, until meat is browned on the outside and no longer pink on the inside.

- Ground turkey sloppy joes served open-faced on multigrain bread.

- Lean beef or ground turkey meatloaf (I use whole-grain bread crumbs).

- Spicy shrimp. Just sauté and serve in a sauce made from a 14.5-ounce can crushed tomatoes, fresh basil, garlic, and ½ tsp. crushed red pepper.

- Soba noodles in a peanut sauce. I make the sauce with ½ cup chicken broth, 2 Tbsp. reduced-fat creamy peanut butter, and 1 Tbsp. each dark brown sugar, low-sodium soy sauce, and fresh lime juice. Just cook the noodles and mix in stir-fry veggies. Toss and serve.

- Asparagus frittata. I love serving this during the hot summer months, because it's light, quick, and easy! I cook up some shallots and asparagus first in a frying pan with a little olive oil, then add the beaten eggs (six in total: one whole egg, five egg whites) and cook till just set. Then I sprinkle shredded low-fat mozzarella cheese on top and toss in the broiler for 4–6 minutes at 400°F, till the cheese is melted and lightly browned. Yum!

cLEAN Momma Pop Quiz: What Kind of Eater Are You?

It's important to understand the how and why of your eating habits so you can live a cLEAN life. Once you recognize your tendencies and triggers, you can sidestep them before they get you! We all eat for various reasons: stress, comfort, pleasure, even boredom. Answer the following statements honestly, and you'll have a clearer picture of what motivates you to munch.

1. Are you a stress eater?

_____ When faced with a tough problem, I reach for the Ben & Jerry's or a bag of chips.

_____ When my kids make me crazy, I deserve something sweet.

_____ My in-laws are coming for the weekend. Time to bake some cupcakes!

If you answered TRUE to most/all of the above, you eat to relieve or avoid uncomfortable feelings. Find another way to blow off steam that doesn't involve bingeing. I highly recommend doing some quick cardio (sweat and get your heart really pumping!). You can exorcise your demons with exercise!

2. Are you a mindless muncher?

_____ When watching *The Real Housewives*, I run to the fridge during commercials.

_____ I keep candy at my desk at work and nibble while I type.

_____ I eat out of the box/bag; who needs to wash another plate?

If you answered TRUE to most/all of the above, you eat unconsciously throughout the day/night, never aware of how much and how often you're consuming food or if it's healthy or not. Keep track of what you eat during the day in a food journal. It will make you much more mindful of what's going in your mouth. And when you eat, take a break from work or TV and pull up a chair at a table. Put your food on a plate, chew it, and let yourself digest and register that you're full.

3. Are you a social eater?

_____ If the waiter brings around the dessert cart, I have to have a sweet . . . or two.

_____ I'll indulge at a party or on the holidays . . . it's a celebration, after all!

_____ Meeting of my book club tonight: chips, dips, and margaritas for me!

If you answered TRUE to most/all of the above, you feel that any occasion with friends or loved ones is a free pass to pig out. A better solution: you can eat anything, but in moderation. And don't drink too much. Not only is a glass of alcohol full of empty calories, but when you're buzzed, you'll be more vulnerable to eating anything that isn't nailed down.

4. Are you an "on the run" eater?

_____ I grab a Pop-Tart or a doughnut while racing out to carpool.

_____ For lunch, I eat whatever is fast and easy—a Fatburger is fine by me.

_____ The kids and hubby are out to dinner and a movie—so I'll just order Chinese takeout. Why cook?

If you answered TRUE to most/all of the above, you think you're too busy to eat healthy—so the staples of your diet are often processed foods from the drive-through window and the vending machine. Cut up veggies, fruits, and high-protein, low-calorie snacks and stash them in your fridge and purse. Prethink your most hectic days and plan ahead of time what you'll eat.

5. Are you an emotional eater?

_____ My overbearing boss just criticized my work. I need a Snickers baaaaaad!

_____ My fight with the hubby over our finances often leads to a Frito-Lay feast.

_____ My kids are at sleepaway camp for the first time. Maybe a caramel macchiato will make me miss them less?

If you answered TRUE to most/all of the above, you react to strong emotions—such as anger, frustration, sadness, even joy—by reaching for food. Think before you eat. Note how you're feeling and really consider your craving: is it physical (i.e., you're hungry) or emotional (i.e., you're trying to fill a void that's not in your tummy!)?

5

Thirty Days of cLEAN Eating: The Intense Plan to Get You *Really* Losing!

cLEAN Momma Says ... Do you eat to live, or live to eat? Think of your food as fuel. Would you put gas in your car ... or diet soda?

YOUR CHAPTER 5 LAUNDRY LIST

- Embrace your cLEAN new way of eating.
- Curb your cravings for junk food.
- Refine your palate and increase your energy with delicious new foods.

NOW THAT YOU'VE GOTTEN A TASTE for what cLEAN eating is all about, it's time to crank it up. This is a lifestyle change. Your body will thank you for it; it will run more efficiently and you'll have more energy, more stamina, and fewer mood swings. I like two things about this plan: first of all, it's simple. I'm not counting calories, weighing my food, or adding up points. (I really suck at math!) Second, it gives me the ability to make my own choices: you choose one from each column (breakfast, lunch, dinner) and two or three snacks (mid-morning, mid-afternoon, late night) each day.

For a lot of people, the key to sustainable weight loss is taking out the refined carbs (and for fastest weight loss, most of the carbs in the form of sugars and starches, whether they're refined or not). Sample some of the recipes (they're delicious!) and work your way up, day by day, to this new way of eating. You won't need junk food when you eat cLEAN food.

Stephanie Lecovin, who gave me my wake-up call, has had such an impact on how I think about food and dieting. She taught me some invaluable lessons! When we eat to fill up, we are less conscious about what we are choosing to fill up with. Sure, bread, cookies, pizza, wine . . . they're yummy! Eat them, but with awareness and within reason. The key is to *fuel* our bodies, not simply to *fill* them. We all want to look great, but looking great on just the outside doesn't cut it. Steph taught me by looking great on the inside, we will effortlessly look great on the outside. Not only will the weight fall off, but your hair, skin, nails, wrinkles, and so on will all look fab! And your heart, organs, cells, and guts will look pretty good too!

Many of the following recipes are from Steph (www.nutritionhousecalls.com). They do more than just fill you up; they fuel you! I hope you enjoy them as much as I do.

THE HAPPY HIPPIE: QUINOA WITH WALNUTS AND BERRIES

Quinoa (*keen-wah*) is an ancient grain from South America. It is packed with nutrients and is also a complete protein! Quinoa has a natural coating called saponin that repels insects and birds and can create a bitter taste. Rinsing the uncooked quinoa with warm water removes the saponin.

MAKES 4 SERVINGS

1 cup quinoa (available in bulk or packaged at many markets and health food stores)

Pinch sea salt

1¾ cups water

6 Tbsp. chopped walnuts

1 cup blueberries (or raspberries, strawberries, blackberries, or other berries)

Maple syrup (if desired)

Rinse quinoa well with warm water and drain. Place the rinsed quinoa, salt, and water in a medium saucepan. Bring to a boil, reduce heat to low, cover and let simmer for 15–20 minutes, or until all the water is absorbed. While quinoa is simmering, toast the walnuts on a cookie sheet in the oven at 350°F for 10–12 minutes (or cook them in a small skillet on the stove over low heat, constantly stirring the nuts to avoid burning). When the quinoa is cooked, fluff with a fork and toss in walnuts. Place in bowls and top with the berries. Drizzle with maple syrup, if desired.

SUPER SMOOTHIE

This smoothie is packed with antioxidants. It's a healthy and delicious way to start your day!

MAKES 1 SERVING

½ large peeled banana, frozen or fresh, broken into chunks

½ cup berries, frozen or fresh

½–1 cup water (start with ½ cup and add more if you prefer a thinner consistency)

2 tsp. nut butter (peanut, almond, or cashew)

¼ cup fresh, packed spinach leaves or other dark, leafy green (e.g., chard or kale), thick stems removed

2 tsp. ground flaxseed and/or hempseed

Place all ingredients in a blender. Blend on high speed until the consistency is smooth. Pour into a glass, serve, and enjoy! The temperature of the smoothie is best if either the banana chunks or the berries are frozen. If neither is frozen, you may add an ice cube to the blender. If additional sweetness is desired, add 1 tsp. local honey or ¼ cup cloudy apple juice. If additional protein is desired, add protein powder (whey, rice, hemp, or soy) or organic plain yogurt.

Recipe by Stephanie Lecovin

FLOURLESS HONEY-ALMOND MUFFINS

Do you know the Muffin Man? I wish I did. What I *do* know is that my family loves muffins, but my thighs don't. If you want a nutritious, guilt-free muffin, however, try these gluten-free, healthy, fiber-filled balls of yum.

MAKES 9 MUFFINS (SERVING SIZE = 1 MUFFIN)

Muffin cups

4 large eggs at room temperature, separated

⅓ cup honey (preferably local)

1 tsp. vanilla extract

½ tsp. baking soda

½ tsp. sea salt

⅛ tsp. ground cinnamon (if desired)

1¾ cups almond meal

½ medium carrot, shredded

½ medium zucchini, shredded

⅓ cup dark chocolate chips (if desired)

Preheat the oven to 325°F. Place 9 muffin cups inside a muffin tin. Beat the egg yolks, honey, vanilla, baking soda, sea salt, and cinnamon in a large bowl with an electric mixer on medium speed until well combined. Add the almond meal, carrot, and zucchini, and beat on low speed until combined. Stir in the chocolate chips (with a rubber spatula), if using. In a separate, medium bowl (and with a clean mixer), beat the egg whites until white and foamy (1–2 minutes). Do not beat for so long that they hold peaks. Gently fold the egg whites into the almond-meal batter with a rubber spatula. Mix until combined, then pour the batter into the muffin cups (fill the cups about ¾ full). Bake for approximately 17 minutes. The muffins should be well formed but still very moist (and slightly browned on top). Allow the muffins to cool for 5–10 minutes.

Recipe by Stephanie Lecovin

DR. GEOFF'S PANCAKES

These gluten-free, dairy-free pancakes are high in protein and taste great, even to those who eat gluten and dairy! Top with berries for extra antioxidants.

MAKES 12 PANCAKES

4 large eggs, plus 3 large egg whites

½ cup certified organic, gluten-free oats

1 cup raw walnuts

2 medium bananas

1 tsp. vanilla extract

½ tsp. cinnamon

coconut oil

fruit, honey, pure maple syrup, or yogurt for garnish

In a blender, combine the eggs and egg whites, oats, walnuts, bananas, vanilla extract, and cinnamon. Blend until smooth. Heat a nonstick pan on medium-high heat. Add enough coconut oil to generously coat the pan. When it's hot (but not smoking), pour the pancake batter onto the pan in 3- to 4-inch rounds. Cook for approximately 1 minute, or until golden brown. Flip the pancakes over and brown the other side (for about another minute). Top with your favorite fruit, honey, pure maple syrup, or yogurt.

Recipe by Stephanie Lecovin

SNACK

- Avocado with fresh lime juice and sea salt

- Berries (or any fresh fruit) and a handful of nuts or plain yogurt

- Celery or apples with peanut butter or almond butter

- Deli turkey (antibiotic-, hormone-, and nitrate-free) wrapped around apple slices

- Edamame (lightly salted soybeans you can enjoy hot or cold)

- Hard-boiled egg and carrots or snap peas

- Mary's Gone Crackers with wild smoked salmon

- Pumpkin seeds (toasted and salted, if desired)

- Tomatoes, minced garlic, extra virgin olive oil, balsamic vinegar, and chopped basil (fresh mozzarella cheese optional)

- Trail mix with almonds, cashews, walnuts, and dark chocolate chips or dried cranberries

- Veggies (carrots, jicama, celery) with hummus

Courtesy of Stephanie Lecovin

PEANUT BUTTER BALLS

While these high-energy balls are decadent enough for dessert, they're healthy enough for a snack! See the Happy Hippie recipe (page 64) for more information about how to cook quinoa.

MAKES 12–15 SERVINGS OF TWO BALLS EACH

1½ cups natural peanut butter (or any sort of nut butter, such as almond, cashew, etc.)

½ cup unsweetened, shredded coconut

½ tsp. sea salt

3 Tbsp. sesame seeds

2 Tbsp. ground flaxseed

2 tsp. vanilla extract

2 Tbsp. honey

1 cup cooked brown rice or quinoa, cooled to room temperature

2 cups dark chocolate chips (optional)

In a medium glass or ceramic bowl, combine the peanut butter, coconut, salt, sesame seeds, ground flaxseed, vanilla extract, and honey. Mix with a spoon until thoroughly combined.

Add rice or quinoa to the peanut butter mixture. Stir until thoroughly mixed.

Line a cookie sheet with parchment paper. Scoop 1 Tbsp. of the dough into your hands and, using your fingers, shape it into a ball. Do this with all of the dough, placing the balls on the parchment-lined cookie sheet. Once the cookie sheet is full, place it in the fridge to chill for at least 1 hour. Melt the chocolate chips in a double boiler until fully melted.

Remove the balls from the fridge and roll them in the chocolate. Use tongs to remove the chocolate-covered balls, one by one, and place them again on the parchment-lined cookie sheet. When the cookie sheet is filled, return it to the fridge and chill until the chocolate has hardened, about 1 hour.

Recipe by Stephanie Lecovin

TASTY TORTILLA CHIPS

These tortilla chips are so delicious that you may think twice before getting store-bought chips next time. Serve with salsa, guacamole, or a bean-based salad.

SERVES 2–4

6 corn tortillas, preferably sprouted corn

2 Tbsp. canola or walnut oil

1 lime, juiced

sea salt, to taste

chili powder, to taste

Preheat the oven to 400°F. Stack the tortillas on a cutting board and cut into triangles (like cutting a pizza). Place the tortilla triangles on a cookie sheet. Drizzle oil onto the tortillas and evenly distribute by tossing them with your hands. Squeeze the fresh lime onto the tortillas along with salt to taste and toss again. Spread evenly on the cookie sheet (making sure they do not overlap) and bake, uncovered, for 10–12 minutes. They can burn quickly, so stay close to the oven!

Recipe by Stephanie Lecovin

GUACAMOLE

I serve this satisfying, easy-to-make dip with the Tasty Tortilla Chips or carrots. It is also a delicious topping for burgers.

2 ripe avocados, peeled, pitted, and diced

1 clove garlic, crushed and minced

1 lime, juiced

sea salt, to taste

½ tsp. finely diced jalapeño, seeds and pith removed (optional)

Mash the avocado in a medium bowl. Mash more for a creamier consistency, less for a chunkier guacamole. Add the garlic, lime juice, and salt, adjusting the amounts based on your personal taste.

Recipe by Stephanie Lecovin

BEAN AND KALE SCRAMBLE

If you ask me, kale is bitter, and if you're not careful, that could be a turn-off. Here's how to make it yummy, because it's so damn good for you!

MAKES 4 SERVINGS

1 tsp. extra virgin olive oil

1 large onion, finely chopped

2 cups Great Northern beans or white beans (cooked or canned), drained and rinsed

¼ cup chopped dill

5 cups chopped kale, stems removed

1 lemon, juiced

1–2 Tbsp. water

2 Tbsp. tamari

1 Tbsp. prepared mustard

In a large skillet, heat the oil over medium heat. Add the onion and sauté for 3 minutes. Add the cooked beans and dill; sauté for another 3 minutes. Add the remaining ingredients and sauté for 5 minutes. Stir occasionally. Serve hot or at room temperature.

Recipe by Stephanie Lecovin

FRESH CRANBERRY-AVOCADO SALSA

Cleansing cranberries and the healthy fats in avocados give this fun salsa a surprising tartness and anti-inflammatory properties.

MAKES 8 SERVINGS

1 Tbsp. fresh lime juice

2 Tbsp. honey

1 minced jalapeño (seeds and membrane removed for less heat)

¼ cup chopped red onion

2 ripe avocados, diced

¾ cup fresh, halved cranberries, drained well on paper towels

2 Tbsp. chopped cilantro

sea salt and freshly ground black pepper, to taste

In a large bowl, whisk together the lime juice and honey. Add the jalapeño and red onion. Toss to combine. Add the remaining ingredients and mix gently. Serve with Tasty Tortilla Chips (page 70) or brown rice, or try it as a sandwich topping.

Recipe by Stephanie Lecovin

GARLIC CHICKPEAS AND GREENS

Chickpeas, also known as garbanzo beans, are high in folate. This recipe also contains folate-rich mustard greens, which give this simple dish almost 90 percent of the daily recommended amount. Mustard greens are grown year-round, so make this nutritious recipe anytime.

MAKES 4 SERVINGS

2 Tbsp. extra virgin olive oil

6 cloves garlic, crushed and minced

1 lb. trimmed mustard greens or another green, e.g., Swiss chard, kale, or escarole, coarsely chopped

sea salt and freshly ground black pepper, to taste

1 cup low-sodium chicken broth

2 (15-oz.) cans chickpeas, drained

Heat a skillet over medium heat. Add the olive oil and garlic. Sauté the garlic for 2 minutes, then add the greens. Briefly wilt the greens in the garlic oil, then season with salt and pepper. Add the chicken broth to the pan. Bring the broth to a soft boil. Cover the pan, reduce the heat to a simmer, and cook the greens 7–8 minutes in the broth. Uncover the pan and add the chickpeas. Adjust seasoning to taste.

Recipe by Stephanie Lecovin

LENTIL AND GREEN OLIVE SALAD

When I heard lentils were such an amazing superfood, I had to try them. They are high in nutrition and low in cost. One word: yum.

MAKES 4 SERVINGS

½ lb. brown or green lentils

1 small onion, peeled

1 garlic clove, peeled

1 bay leaf

sea salt and freshly ground black pepper, to taste

1 cup pitted and coarsely chopped imported green olives

1 red bell pepper, cut into long, thin strips, then in thirds (so they are bite-size)

⅓ cup extra virgin olive oil

3 Tbsp. fresh lemon juice

bitter greens such as arugula, chicory, frisée, radicchio, or tender dandelions

zest of ½ lemon, cut into fine julienne strips

1 Tbsp. minced flat-leaf parsley

Pick the lentils over carefully to get rid of any small stones or grit. Rinse them under running water. Place them in a saucepan over medium heat. Add 3 cups cool water. Add the onion, garlic, bay leaf, salt, and pepper, and bring to a boil. When the water is boiling, turn down the heat, cover the lentils, and simmer for about 30 minutes, or until the lentils are thoroughly cooked and tender. When the lentils are done, drain them, discarding the vegetables, and mix, while still warm, with the olives, red pepper, olive oil, and lemon juice. Taste and adjust the seasonings, if necessary. Serve the lentils piled on a bed of bitter greens. Garnish with the julienne strips of lemon zest and minced parsley.

Recipe by Stephanie Lecovin

MANGO AND BEAN SALAD WITH CORN TORTILLAS

This colorful salad is packed with inflammation-fighting fruits and vegetables.

MAKES 8 PORTIONS (½ CUP EACH)

4 large ripe mangoes, peeled, pitted, and cubed

1 cup cubed pineapple

½ medium cucumber, seeded and sliced

¼ cup finely chopped red bell pepper

4 small green onions, thinly sliced

1 (15-oz.) can black beans, rinsed and drained

HONEY-LIME DRESSING

2 Tbsp. extra virgin olive oil

1 Tbsp. honey

3–4 tsp. lime juice

1 tsp. grated lime rind

1 Tbsp. wine vinegar

2 Tbsp. water

½ tsp. dried mint leaves or 1½ tsp. chopped mint

pinch of salt

8 corn tortillas (preferably sprouted corn)

Whisk all the dressing ingredients together in a medium bowl. Set aside. Combine the mangoes, pineapple, cucumber, bell pepper, green onions, and black beans in another bowl; drizzle with the lime dressing and toss gently. Serve with the corn tortillas.

Recipe by Stephanie Lecovin

MEDITERRANEAN TUNA SALAD

Tuna is great for weight loss: high in protein and huge in omega-3 fatty acids, which are so good for your body. This recipe will make even the pickiest eaters love tuna!

MAKES 4 SERVINGS

4 (6-oz.) cans chunk light tuna, drained well

1 (14-oz.) can artichoke hearts, drained and coarsely chopped

½ cup chopped red bell pepper

¾ cup coarsely chopped Greek olives

½ small red onion, minced

¼ cup minced Italian parsley

¼ cup minced basil

2 garlic cloves, minced

1 tsp. dried oregano or 1 Tbsp. fresh oregano

1 cup mayonnaise

3 Tbsp. lemon juice

freshly ground black pepper

In a large bowl, combine the tuna, artichoke hearts, red pepper, olives, onion, parsley, basil, garlic, oregano, mayonnaise, lemon juice, and pepper and mix until well combined. Serve the salad on mixed greens with diced avocado (and any other colorful veggies desired).

LEMON CHICKEN

Chicken can get boring, but when I make this dish for my family, my kids gobble it down! This low-calorie, low-fat meal is rich in taste.

MAKES 4 SERVINGS

8–10 boneless and skinless chicken tenderloin breasts

1 tsp. sea salt

freshly ground pepper, to taste

5 Tbsp. lemon juice, divided

¼ cup flour

3 tsp. extra virgin olive oil, divided

1 cup chopped onion or shallots

½ cup dry white wine

1 (14-oz.) can low-sodium chicken broth

⅓ cup low-fat sour cream

Using a mallet or a heavy pan, pound the chicken breasts between two pieces of wax paper so they become nice and thin. Season the pieces with salt and pepper, making sure to coat all sides. Drizzle them with 2 Tbsp. of the lemon juice. Then coat the chicken with the flour and place it in a baking dish.

Heat 2 tsp. of the olive oil in a large nonstick skillet over medium-high heat. Lightly brown the chicken, about 3 minutes on each side. Set the chicken aside, covered to keep it warm.

Heat the remaining tsp. of the oil in the same pan over medium-high heat. Add the onion or shallots and sauté until they are brown. Sprinkle with some of the flour and add 3 more Tbsp. of the lemon juice, the wine, and the chicken broth. Season with a tiny bit of salt and bring to a boil. (Remember to keep stirring.)

Return the chicken to the pan and reduce the heat. Let the chicken simmer for about 7 minutes. Add the sour cream, and stir until the sauce is creamy and smooth.

TUSCAN WHITE BEAN SOUP

This is a flavorful soup with a hearty, smooth texture and the taste of fresh herbs, combined with the rich taste of tomatoes and garlic.

MAKES 8 SERVINGS

2 cups white beans, soaked overnight (canned is also fine)

4 bay leaves

2 Tbsp. minced rosemary

10 cups cold water

2 Tbsp. extra virgin olive oil

1–2 Tbsp. sea salt

1 yellow onion, diced

¼ tsp. crushed red pepper

8–10 cloves garlic, minced

4 ripe Roma tomatoes, seeded and diced

1 small bunch fresh kale, thick stems removed

1 Tbsp. balsamic vinegar

1 tsp. freshly ground black pepper

Soak the beans in water overnight, for at least 8 hours. Drain and rinse the beans and place them in a 4-qt. pot with the bay leaves, 2 tsp. of the minced rosemary, and the cold water. Bring the mixture to a boil and then reduce the heat and let simmer for 15 minutes. Skim the top of the water and discard; add 1 Tbsp. of the olive oil and continue to simmer the remaining mixture for 45–60 minutes. Add 2 tsp. of the salt to the beans when they've finished cooking and are tender.

Heat the remaining Tbsp. of the olive oil in a separate pot and add the onion, 1 tsp. of the salt, and the crushed red pepper. Sauté the mixture until the onions are golden and soft. Add the garlic and the remaining rosemary, and cook for 5–10 minutes on medium heat.

Next, add the beans and their cooking liquid to the onion and garlic mixture. Begin to simmer all the ingredients while adding the tomatoes. Let simmer for 20 minutes.

While the mixture is simmering, wash and cut the stems off the kale, tear the leaves into bite-size pieces, and add to the soup within the last 5–10 minutes of cooking. Season the soup to taste with the balsamic vinegar, black pepper, and remaining salt. Serve immediately.

Recipe by Stephanie Lecovin

-ETHIOPIAN CHICKPEA STEW

I dare you to look up the health benefits of garbanzo beans. Try this yummy soup, and you'll feel full, fueled, and healthy!

SERVES 6

1 tsp. sweet paprika

1 tsp. sea salt

½ tsp. ground allspice

½ tsp. freshly ground black pepper

½ tsp. ground cardamom

½ tsp. ground cloves

½ tsp. ground coriander

⅛–¼ tsp. cayenne

½ tsp. ground ginger

2 (15-oz.) cans no-salt-added chickpeas, rinsed and drained

3 Tbsp. extra virgin olive oil

2 cloves garlic, minced

1 medium red onion, chopped

One 1-inch piece fresh ginger, peeled and finely chopped

1 (8-oz.) can no-salt-added tomato sauce

1 qt. low-sodium vegetable broth

1 lb. red potatoes, cut into 1-inch chunks

4 carrots, peeled and cut into 1-inch chunks

Preheat the oven to 450°F. Stir together the paprika, salt, allspice, black pepper, cardamom, cloves, coriander, cayenne, and ginger in a small bowl; set the spice mixture aside.

Toss the chickpeas with 1 Tbsp. of the oil on a large, rimmed baking sheet and spread them out in a single layer. Roast the chickpeas, stirring occasionally, until somewhat dried out and just golden brown, 16–18 minutes; set aside. Meanwhile, heat the remaining 2 Tbsp. of oil in a medium pot over medium heat. Add the garlic, onion, and chopped ginger, and cook, stirring occasionally, until very soft and golden brown, 8–10 minutes. Stir in the reserved spice mixture and continue cooking, stirring constantly, until the spices are toasted and very fragrant, about 2 minutes. Stir in the tomato sauce and cook 2 minutes more.

Stir in the broth, potatoes, carrots, and reserved chickpeas, and bring to a boil. Reduce the heat to medium-low, cover, and simmer until the potatoes and carrots are just tender, about 20 minutes. Uncover the pot and simmer until the stew is thickened and the potatoes and carrots are very tender, about 25 minutes more. Ladle the stew into bowls and serve.

If you're in a hurry, omit roasting the chickpeas and simply add them to the stew after they've been rinsed and drained.

Recipe by Stephanie Lecovin

PITA POCKET STEAK AND SALAD STUFFER

This recipe is really healthy and really simple—a great dinner on the go.

¼ cup lemon juice

1 tsp. mustard

1 tsp. maple syrup

A pinch each of salt and pepper

¼ tsp. garlic salt

1 lb. *very* lean steak (I like it on the thin side, about 1-inch thick)

2 cups chopped spinach leaves

1 cup chopped romaine lettuce

1 large tomato, diced

1 cucumber, diced

Eight 4-inch whole wheat pitas

Preheat the broiler. In a small bowl, whisk together the lemon juice, mustard, maple syrup, salt and pepper, and garlic salt.

Place the steak in a broiling pan that's not too deep, and pour half of the marinade on it. Let the steak marinate for 15–20 minutes while you finish preparing the rest of the meal. Make sure you flip the steak so it gets coated on all sides.

In a separate bowl, combine the spinach, romaine, tomato, cucumber, and the rest of the marinade. Toss the salad really well so it's well coated. (I like adding a bit more lemon juice.)

Broil the steak for 5–8 minutes on each side, depending on how you like it cooked. Allow it to cool on a cutting board, and then cut it into thin slices.

Mix the meat with the salad and toss. Stuff the pitas with the steak and salad mixture and enjoy. My kids love it when I warm up the pitas before I stuff them—15 seconds in the microwave is plenty.

STEAK AND SHRIMP STIR-FRY

I like this low-calorie, low-carb recipe, because it's yummy and super easy, and my friends are impressed when they come over. It also takes less than 30 minutes! (When I make it for my kids, I don't make it spicy, but I add a kick of spice for my portion.)

MAKES 4 SERVINGS

¼ cup rice wine

1 Tbsp. Trader Joe's Soyaki or a light teriyaki sauce

1½ Tbsp. oyster sauce

2 tsp. cornstarch

4 tsp. olive oil, divided

¾ lb. very lean steak, very thinly sliced

sea salt and freshly ground black pepper, to taste

¼–½ tsp. crushed red pepper (If I make this for my kids, I leave out the red pepper but add a dash of cayenne pepper to my own portion.)

15 raw shrimp (I get the frozen kind at Trader Joe's, which saves time since they are already peeled.)

1 cup chopped baby bok choy (cut into 1-inch pieces)

½ cup mandarin orange pieces (I use the canned ones and pour out the juice.)

In a small bowl, mix the rice wine, Soyaki or teriyaki, oyster sauce, and cornstarch.

In a large wok or skillet, heat 2 tsp. of the olive oil over high heat. When the oil is hot, add the steak, salt and pepper, and the crushed red pepper. Cook the meat, stirring, until it browns, about 2 minutes. Add the shrimp and cook for another 2 minutes until it becomes pink. Remove the meat and shrimp and set them aside in a separate bowl.

In the same wok or skillet, heat 2 more tsp. of the olive oil over medium-high heat. Add the bok choy and cook, stirring until it wilts, about 2 minutes. Add the mandarin oranges, and cook for another 2 minute.

Stir in the cornstarch mixture along with the beef and shrimp. Cook until the sauce thickens, about a minute.

Serve with brown rice and a side of veggies if you wish. (My kids like to eat it with steamed broccoli).

SALMON CAKES

If you want to impress your guests, serve this! Little will they know how easy it is to make and how healthy it is to eat.

1 Tbsp. plus 2–3 tsp. extra virgin olive oil

½ red onion, finely chopped

1½–2 lbs. wild salmon, skin and bones removed, cut into large chunks

1 egg

1 tsp. sea salt

freshly ground black pepper, to taste

¼ cup mayonnaise

1 Tbsp. dill (fresh or dried), or more, if desired

Heat the olive oil in a sauté pan. Add the onions and cook on low to medium heat until the onions are brown. Remove from the heat and place in a medium or large bowl. Put the salmon in a food processor, add the egg, salt, and pepper, and process until thoroughly combined, about 10 seconds (don't overmix, or the salmon will get mushy). Add the salmon mixture to the bowl and mix until combined with the onion. Form the mixture into patties. Add more olive oil (2–3 tsp.) to the pan and cook the patties on medium heat until browned on each side and cooked through, 2–3 minutes per side.

In a small bowl, mix the mayonnaise and dill until thoroughly combined. Serve the salmon cakes with a dollop of dill mayo on the side.

Recipe by Stephanie Lecovin

NO-BAKE CHOCOLATE BROWNIES

1 cup raw walnut pieces

1 cup medjool dates, pits removed

½ cup cacao powder

pinch sea salt

1–2 Tbsp. raw cacao nibs, or to taste

Place the walnuts in a food processor and grind for a couple of seconds to form a coarse flour. While the machine is running, add the pitted dates, cacao powder, and salt, processing until a moist, crumblike dough has formed.

Spread the dough into an 8 × 8–inch pan, sprinkle with cacao nibs, and press firmly into a solid brownie layer. Cut into bite-size squares and serve. You can also press and roll the brownie dough into small balls to make brownie bites.

Recipe by Stephanie Lecovin

For a sweet tooth . . .

It's okay to indulge a few times a week. Giving in to a craving once in a while (remember: moderation!) means you'll be less likely to ditch your cLEAN eating plan and binge. I am partial to hot cocoa with mini-marshmallows (I love to sip and savor it slooooowly). Stephanie recommends:

- ¼ to ½ oz. high-quality dark chocolate (at least 68% cacao)
- Dipping strawberries in dark chocolate would be fine, too

CHOCOLATE BARK

This recipe is not only packed with antioxidants but also tastes outrageously decadent.

MAKES 3 MEDIUM-SIZE PIECES

3 Tbsp. canola or walnut oil

6 Tbsp. pure maple syrup

2 cups raw pecans

½ tsp. sea salt

¼ tsp. cayenne (less if you can't stand the heat)

½ tsp. cinnamon

½ tsp. nutmeg

3 cups dark chocolate (at least 70% cacao)

Preheat the oven to 400°F. In a large skillet, heat the oil and maple syrup until bubbling. Add the pecans and stir until they are well coated, then mix in the salt and seasonings. Cook for 4 minutes, then remove the pan from the heat.

Place the nuts on a parchment-lined baking sheet. Place the sheet in the oven and roast for 4 minutes. Remove from the oven and cool completely.

In a separate saucepan, melt the chocolate over very low heat, stirring often. Pour the chocolate into a parchment-lined 13 × 9–inch glass dish or onto a larger baking sheet (depending on whether you want the bark to be thicker or thinner). Break up the pecans and sprinkle over the chocolate. Using a spatula, spread the mixture evenly. Allow the bark to sit out until set, 1–2 hours. Break it apart into chunks.

FABULOUS FRUIT CRISP

Almost any fruit may be used in this recipe, including berries, apples, pears, mangoes . . . even bananas! Frozen fruit works just as well as fresh. This is an easy recipe for kids, so get them involved!

MAKES 8 SERVINGS

1 cup rolled oats

½ cup flour (whole-wheat pastry flour, rice flour, etc.)

½ tsp. sea salt

¼ cup canola oil (or another cold-pressed vegetable oil)

¼ cup pure maple syrup

⅓ cup chopped nuts (cashews, walnuts, or pecans work well)

2 Tbsp. water

2 Tbsp. maple syrup

1 tsp. cinnamon

¼ tsp. nutmeg (optional)

2 tsp. pure vanilla extract

5 cups chopped fruit (if using berries, leave them whole)

Preheat the oven to 350°F. Mix the oats, flour, and salt together in a bowl. Add the oil and maple syrup; mix well. Stir in the nuts and set aside. In a small bowl, combine the water, syrup, spices, and vanilla extract; set aside. Place the chopped fruit in a lightly oiled pie pan or an 8 × 8–inch baking dish. Pour the liquid mixture over the fruit and toss gently. Spoon the oat-nut mixture evenly on top of the fruit. Cover and bake for 45 minutes. Uncover and bake 15 minutes more to crisp the topping.

Recipe by Stephanie Lecovin

RAW CHOCOLATE MACAROONS

These macaroons would make Bubbie proud!

MAKES ABOUT 20 MACAROONS

3 cups dried, unsweetened coconut flakes

1½ cups raw cacao powder

1 cup pure maple syrup

⅓ cup coconut oil, melted

1 Tbsp. pure vanilla extract

½ tsp. sea salt

Place all the ingredients in a large bowl and stir well to combine. Using a small ice cream scoop, your hands, or a big tablespoon, make rounds of the dough and put them onto a plate or cutting board to freeze.

FOR BLOND MACAROONS: Replace the cocoa powder in the recipe with an equal amount of fine almond flour. They are just as delish!

Recipe by Stephanie Lecovin

cLEAN Momma Pop Quiz: Are You Ready for Change?

Losing weight and keeping it off is not about the latest crash diet in the tabloids. It depends on making permanent lifestyle changes—that includes eating healthy and exercising, as well as owning up to the things that are holding you back. Knowing that you need to make changes in your life and actually *doing* it are very different. Answer these questions honestly:

_____ Have you dealt with all the major distractions in your life (e.g., marital problems, stress, financial worries, etc.)? Overhauling your eating habits is a challenge—you don't want any other major issues standing in your way.

_____ Do you have a realistic weight-loss goal? As I've said before, this is a lifelong process, not a quick fix. How much do you want to lose, and what is a reasonable amount of time to do that in? It's best to aim for 1 to 2 pounds a week.

_____ Have you dealt with your emotions?

_____ As we've already learned, stress, anxiety, grief, frustration, and boredom can all trigger emotional eating. Are you in a good place emotionally, where you won't be "led astray"?

_____ Do you have the right support?

_____ If you're tempted, who will be there (your mom, sis, BFF, hubby) to help you stay focused and true to your goals?

_____ Are you ready to be responsible for your actions?

_____ Are you willing to do what it takes to cLEAN up your act? Will you keep a log of your eating/exercising? Are you excited about feeling healthy and happy again?

If you answered NO to any of the above, that's okay. You can explore what's holding you back and face those obstacles. Sometimes it's simply a matter of timing. You may have too much going on around you and you're afraid you can't make the leap. Change is scary, sure. But staying in a place where you feel and look terrible . . . that's terrifying. Take one day at a time, one goal at a time.

cLEAN
Body

6
What Is Taskercise?

cLEAN Momma Says ... Every day you have tons of opportunities to fit in exercise. Get lean while you clean ... while you shop ... while you take the kids to school. Get the picture?

YOUR CHAPTER 6 LAUNDRY LIST

- Stop making excuses and start exercising.
- See the benefit of exercise for both mind and body.
- Understand that Taskercise fits into every life and lifestyle.
- Incorporate the Taskercise 25 into your daily schedule.

I hate cleaning. But I also hate having to lie down to zip up my jeans. After popping out a second kid and gaining sixty pounds, I knew I needed to make exercise a priority in my life. But when I took the time to hit the gym three to four times a week for an hour or two a day, it seemed it was always at the expense of a dirty, sticky kitchen, or a mountain of laundry piled up in my closet (I figured if I couldn't *see* the

DOWN AND DIRTY TIP: Toy Story

Have your kids give their toy cars a car wash! Get a cooking pot with some soapy water and a scrubber. Then have your kids take their Matchbox cars to the car wash. Not only can you get rid of all the germy germs and get clean, shiny, like-new toys, but your kids will have a blast doing water play with the car wash!

dirty clothes, they simply weren't there). I could never seem to find the time to have both things in my life: a clean house and a tight tush.

When women tell me, "I have no time to work out," I totally get it. I feel your pain. When you're a frazzled mom, you have not a second to spare to sweat (at least not on purpose!). On the big list of priorities, your spare tire, oversized butt, and saggy arms are way, way down there, somewhere below "shave my legs." Kids come first; life comes second. And even if you are momentarily motivated to join the gym, start a diet, and lose some weight, it's hard to keep up that momentum. Two to three months later, I always went back to my old habits.

That's why I came up with my exercise plan. I call it Taskercising. Why? Because it's about juggling everything you have to get done while sneaking in some great fat-burning, blood-pumping exercises. As I said before, I came up with this brilliant idea after my then two-month-old son, Jack, puked up all over me and my kitchen floor. After I screamed, "Oh my god! Gross!" I threw down my dish towel and used my foot to wipe up the mess while I juggled Jack in my arms. Basically, all I did was smear his puke around on my floor (Sorry! TMI!) but I did feel a burn in my inner thighs.

Eureka! I quickly put Jack in his swing so I could explore this idea further. I threw a couple of damp rags on my kitchen floor with some water and soap and began to use my feet as mops. Since I'd trained as a dancer for over twenty years, form and technique came easy to me. I was soon sweating bullets and my heart was racing. This was an incredible cardio workout! And it was also pretty fun . . . despite the smell.

I was amazed! What other rooms would this work in? That night, while in the bathroom, bathing my kids in the tub, I did the same exercise, mopping my floor. The Rag Drag was born! But my brain didn't stop there. Soon every room and every chore was an opportunity to Taskercise! I could reach, stretch, pump, bend, squat . . . all while doing housework. I thought, "Gee, these containers of bleach are heavy. What if I lifted them like dumbbells for a few reps?" Little by little, I started to incorporate these exercises into my daily routine and build upon them. After only a week, my energy was higher, I felt stronger, and I slept better. I knew I was onto something.

Fast-forward a few months, and I was loving my routine. It was a miracle, a workout that actually worked within my crazy schedule. I would do it every day, everywhere. I was determined to throw my disgusting, oversize sweats into the incinerator and get back into my skinny jeans! With each chore, I remembered what they taught me in ballet: pull up, keep your hips square, kick your legs up, and don't stick your tush out. So I did just that! While I did the dishes, folded laundry, blow-dried my hair, brushed my teeth . . . you get the picture. It became second nature. Without even paying attention or obsessing over working out, I began to drop the pounds. In less than four months, I was thinner and more toned than when I was twenty years old, doing national tours of *A Chorus Line*! And my house? It was clean and organized.

All my mommy friends started hounding me: "Oh my god! What are you doing? How did you get back in shape so fast?" So I showed them. Of course they laughed and completely made fun of me ("Carolyn has finally lost it!"). But that was it; I *had* lost it—I'd lost all that excess weight and bulge. My friends could laugh all they wanted; but then they'd say, "I wish I had your butt." And guess who's Taskercizing now?

Why Exercise?

Aside from the obvious (you're tired of looking like the Pillsbury Dough Mom), working out works wonders for both mind and body.

- **YOU'LL BURN MORE CALORIES. When you get your body moving, you speed up your metabolism. Translation: You're going to burn calories more efficiently and** frequently, so what passes through your lips won't land on your hips. Your metabolism is the way your body processes and uses the food you eat. A recent study showed that the effects of exercising vigorously for forty-five minutes were maintained over the next fourteen hours. That means you can sit on your butt and still burn calories. Love it!

- **YOU'LL BUILD MORE MUSCLE.** Women lose five or six pounds of muscle each decade, starting in their mid-twenties. And when muscle goes down (you guessed it!), fat goes up. You have to exercise to combat this. I'm not talking about bulking up and looking like a female bodybuilder. You just want to tone. Here's a fun fact: every pound of muscle uses about six calories a day just to sustain itself, while each pound of fat burns only two calories daily. So the more muscle you have, the more you burn.

- **IT MAKES YOU HAPPY.** Working out increases your endorphins (aka happy chemicals in your brain), as well as blood flow to your brain and oxygen to your lungs and organs. You simply feel better!

- **IT REDUCES STRESS.** Exercising for just thirty minutes can blow off tension by increasing levels of soothing brain chemicals, such as serotonin, dopamine, and norepinephrine. It's like a natural tonic for your nerves!

- **IT HELPS BEAT THE BLUES.** Studies show that burning off 350 calories three times a week through sustained activity can reduce symptoms of depression as effectively as antidepressants. That may be because exercise appears to stimulate the growth of neurons in certain brain regions damaged by depression.

- **IT BUILDS SELF-CONFIDENCE.** You don't have to see a major change in your body to feel sexier, stronger, and more self-assured. Studies suggest that simply making an effort to exercise every day in some way can improve your body image.

- **IT MAKES YOU SMARTER.** Even mild activity can help keep your brain fit and active, fending off memory loss. Exercise appears to protect the hippocampus, which governs memory and spatial navigation. Researchers even recommend it to reduce the risk of Alzheimer's!

- **IT MAKES YOU LOOK YOUNGER.** Sweat purges your body of toxins that can clog pores and plague your skin with pimples. Exercise also gets blood and oxygen flowing to the skin, carrying nutrients and natural oils to give you a glow and keep wrinkles at bay.

Excuses, Excuses!

Honey, I've heard 'em all . . .

"I DON'T HAVE ENOUGH TIME TO EXERCISE." If you have two or three minutes a day, you can fit in exercise. Run up the stairs instead of taking an elevator. Walk home instead of hopping on the bus. Put your tennis shoes on in the A.M. if you're not going any place fancy schmancy. Every minute is an opportunity to be active. You just have to choose to make the most of your time.

"I'M TOO TIRED TO EXERCISE." I hear ya. There are days I would rather collapse in a heap on the floor instead of doing ten crunches. But here's my little secret: regular exercise actually gives you more energy. The more you move, the less fatigued you'll feel. Anything that strengthens the heart and lungs will boost your oxygen intake. And that means greater stamina.

"I'M TOO OLD/TOO FAT/TOO UNHEALTHY TO START EXERCISING." It's never too late to start exercising. Researchers say that starting a workout program even later in life can greatly improve your health. It can reduce your risk of heart disease, cancer, and other diseases significantly. People can sometimes even control conditions such as diabetes and high blood pressure with weight loss and exercise so they don't need to continue their medications. I like to think of exercise as an insurance policy. If you're concerned about starting a workout (e.g., you have a bad back, knees, etc.), your doctor can help guide you.

"I'LL HURT MYSELF." You're actually *less* likely to hurt yourself if you work out regularly. Exercise increases flexibility and balance (so you're less likely to take a spill). And stronger muscles help support your bones and joints. Translation: less aches and pains.

(continued)

> **"EXERCISE IS BORING."** Not all exercise is boring; everyone can find a physical activity they enjoy. It could be gardening, swimming, tennis, walking your dog. Taskercise is great for people who are "anti-exercise," because you're sneaking it into your daily routine. You won't even realize you're getting a workout; you'll just see the results.

Taskercising 101

Multitasking is what we moms do on a daily basis. Our brains are wired to function this way. We naturally think, "Well, I might as well kill two birds (or three or four!) with one stone . . ." That's why my program works; it's multitasking at its finest. You can clean your house and get in shape simultaneously. And guess what that leaves over: more time for you. More time to breathe, nap, get your nails done. You will never have to make a choice again between taking care of your home and taking care of yourself. Think of them now as one perfect little package. Plus, you don't need a gym membership, fancy weights, or equipment to do this program. Whatever you have around the house will do: dishrags, empty bleach bottles, your vacuum cleaner . . .

What I put together in this chapter is a highly effective interval-training program that meets the needs of beginners as well as the hyperactive (like *moi!*), who prefer a boot-camp approach. The ideas behind the routine are simple: with proper technique, you can sculpt a lean body while you clean. This is not just another workout routine; this is a lifestyle change. It's a change in your habits, the way you carry your body, the way you think and feel.

GETTING STARTED

There are two ways you can approach this workout. The first way is to spread it out through your entire day, while doing daily chores, like washing dishes or cleaning your countertops. Let's call this the "sneak it in" approach. It works around your kids and your life at home. I'll show you exercises you can sneak in while cleaning or doing mundane activities in any room. Try a few, then a few more. You may need to look at the

DOWN AND DIRTY TIP: The Power of the Baby Wipe

I keep baby wipes in almost every room of my house, and my kids are six and nine. They're not just for tiny tushies, ya know. Baby wipes are chemical-free and one of the easiest ways to clean up gook and wipe down dust. You can also use them to blot coffee stains out of your rug or sofa, shine your shoes, even wipe down your BBQ grill!

book at first and study till you familiarize yourself with the exercise. That's okay. I give you permission to cheat. But, eventually, these exercises will feel like second nature to you. You'll be scrubbing pots while doing deep knee-bends!

The second way is more concentrated—let's call it the "revved up" approach. You're going to do my strengthening exercises and sweat for fifteen to twenty minutes a day, three times a week. You'll follow a combination of Taskercises that specially target your trouble areas, such as arms, abs, legs, and butt (see page 145). Once you master the "sneak it in" approach, you may want to amp up your workout, adding in some of these combinations to see results quicker.

Either way requires a commitment: "I will do this. I will stick with it." You'll also be logging your workout (see the chart on page 147), which will help you visualize how much you're getting done. Your log will hold you accountable. I said Taskercise was fun and easy, but you have to work at it. The fat isn't going to fly off you; you have to *move* to see results. You get out of it what you put in. That doesn't mean you have to work out for hours each day. It just means you need to work out smart.

Some things to remember before starting:

- **DOC KNOWS BEST.** Check with your doctor before starting any exercise program.

- **THINK TALL.** Posture and form are very important. Engage, be present, and pay attention to your body. Practice this concept throughout the day, not just when you Taskercise. Imagine a big string connected to your head pulling you up, and every time you slouch, jerk that string. It's amazing how you can change your entire body image within seconds just by correcting your posture. It will lengthen your spine and elongate your muscles so you'll have a stronger frame and core—and will be less likely to pull or strain something.

- **FOCUS AND DON'T RACE THROUGH IT.** When you control each move, you are targeting the muscle group specifically, giving it a better workout. Your dishes won't get done faster if you flap your legs up and down. Make it a rule to hold your position for at least two or three seconds per rep. This helps with core stabilization and strengthens the tummy.

- **EASE INTO THE WORKOUT PLAN.** Just as I advised you to do with the cLEAN Diet, I want you to take the cLEAN Body program one small step at a time. If you're going to try out all of the Taskercises at once, don't do more than a few at a time. A better strategy is to take some time to let yourself get used to them. Don't overdo it! You can also spread out the Taskercises through the day, giving yourself some time between reps to rest up.

THE WARM-UP/PICK-UP

Start with a brisk walk that gradually increases in speed as you move throughout the house, putting your stuff away. Bonus if you have stairs! This is just a great way to wake up your muscles and get your blood circulating to them! Bend over; stretch high; twist and reach. I recommend doing this for five minutes before you begin to Taskercise.

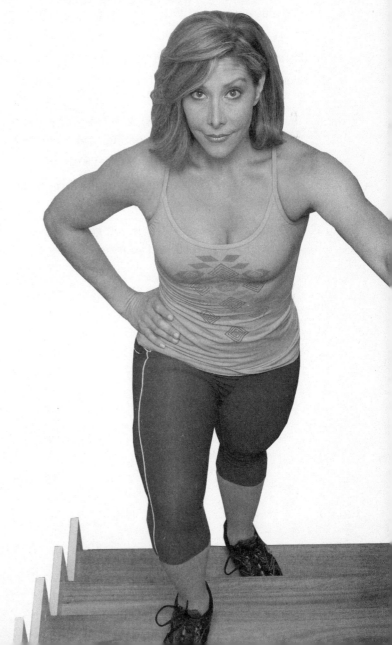

TASKERCISE 1: THE RAG DRAG

The one that started it all! This is your main cardio move. You can multitask while cleaning your floors with this move, or you can also use it for one-minute intervals of short bursts of high intensity between repetitions of the cleaning exercises. The other option for your cardio is to do the cLEAN Momma Rag Drag at the end of your cleaning workout for ten to twelve minutes. Then cool down and stretch.

WHAT YOU NEED: Two damp rags or paper towels to throw down on your floor.
NOTE: If you have carpeting, you can throw down two pieces of cardboard or paper plates and do the same moves.

WHERE TO DO IT: The kitchen, bathroom, anywhere you have a floor that needs washing/waxing/polishing

WHAT IT WORKS: While you get an aerobic workout, you will also tighten your thighs, your tush, and your tummy.

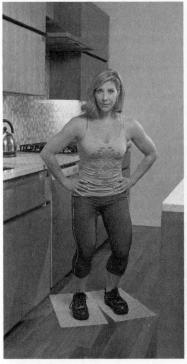
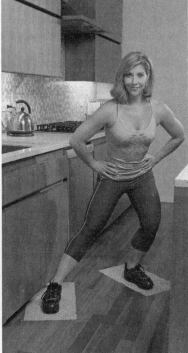
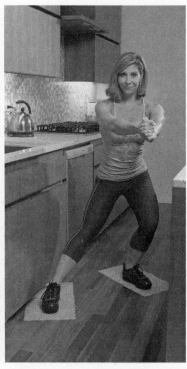

1. Get two damp rags and place them in front of your feet, approximately shoulder-width apart. Step on top of the rags, then lightly bend your knees, keeping your tush tucked in, your spine straight, and your hands on your hips.

2. Start with your right leg, bringing it in and out 5 times, counting down to 1. Bend your left knee. Make sure your knee doesn't go past your toe.

3. As you bring your right foot in and out, put pressure on your working foot, wiping away the gunk on the floor. The resistance is what makes this a great workout.

4. Switch legs and repeat for 5 reps, bringing your left leg in and out 5 times, counting down to 1.

5. Choose another part of your floor, and bring your foot in and out for a 4-count on each leg, counting down to 1 on each leg.

6. Relocate, then do a 3-count on each leg, counting down to 1 on each leg. Repeat this countdown from 5 to 4, 3, 2, 1, and do that 3 times, making your way around the entire floor.

TO REV IT UP: Clasp your hands together instead of putting them on your hips to elevate your heart rate.

TASKERCISE 2: THE RAG DRAG TWIST

WHAT YOU NEED: Two rags or paper towels. Note: if you have carpeting, you can throw down two pieces of cardboard or paper plates and do the same moves.

WHERE TO DO IT: The kitchen, bathroom, anywhere you have a floor that needs washing/waxing/polishing

WHAT IT WORKS: Your waistline, obliques, and back flab

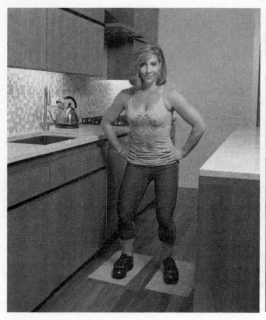
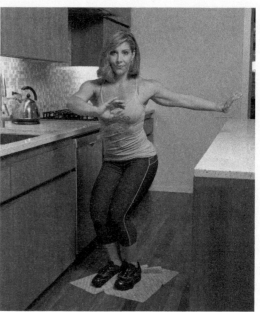

1. Place two damp rags next to each other on the floor, and step one foot onto each rag. Bend your knees and make sure your entire weight is supported by your foot.

2. Bring your feet together. Fully extend your right arm out to the side, and bend your left elbow keeping your arm at boob level as you twist to the left. When you change your twist to the right, extend your left arm out and bend your right elbow. Make sure your arms stay at boob level; this will elevate your heart rate. (Remember to keep your weight on

your foot to really get the most out of this twist, and to really clean those floors!)

3. Keeping your shoulders down and tush tucked in, twist from left to right. Make sure your core is engaged, and your tummy is tucked in.

4. Do the Twist for 30 seconds. If you can, work up to a full minute several times throughout your day.

TASKERCISE 3: TIME PRESS

WHAT YOU NEED: A countertop or a wall

WHERE TO DO IT: At the stove when you're waiting for pasta to boil or by the counter while the microwave is running. I used to do this while changing my kids' diapers!

WHAT IT WORKS: When you're pressed for time, do these time presses to shape your back, your chest, and your arms, as well as tighten your core.

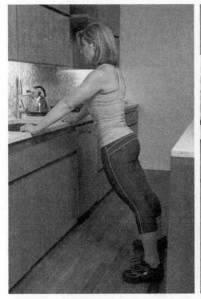
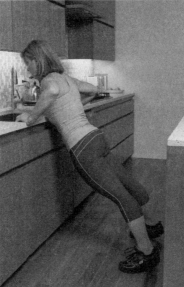
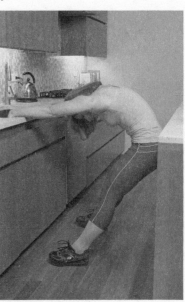

1. Stand with your feet shoulder-width apart, and stand about 2 feet away from your counter or sink.

2. Place your hands on the counter/sink, shoulder-width apart, with your fingertips facing away from your body.

3. Making sure your shoulders are down and your neck and spine are straight, inhale through your nose. As you exhale through and bring your chest to the counter/sink, move your elbows out to the side; do not drop them toward the floor. Then, come back to the

start position. Do two sets of 12–15 reps. It's important to keep your tush tucked under you and tight and your abs engaged. Also, keeping your neck in line with your spine will prevent you from tightening your shoulders.

TO REV IT UP: Hold the last Time Press of the set in a plank position for 15–30 seconds. To do this, instead of coming back up and straightening your arms, stay low with bent elbows, neck in line with spine, back straight and abs tight. Your chest should be about 2

inches from your countertop/sink.

NOTE: It's always important to stretch out after exercise. Its takes only a moment. Hold onto your sink/countertop and pull your tush away while straightening your arms and legs. Lean forward and curl your lower back by imagining your belly button reaching toward your spine.

Hold this position for 20–30 seconds as you inhale through your nose and exhale through your mouth. Relax your neck!

TASKERCISE 4: SUDS ME UP!

WHAT YOU NEED: Sink filled with dirty dishes; dishwashing liquid, sponge

WHERE TO DO IT: Kitchen

WHAT IT WORKS: I like to think of this as my butt-burning, saddlebag-slimming, dish-washing system! You can do this before you load your dishwasher or, if you prefer, stack before drying.

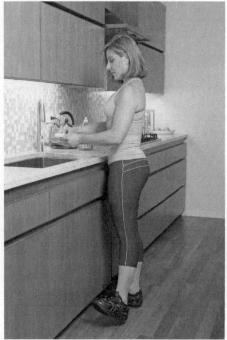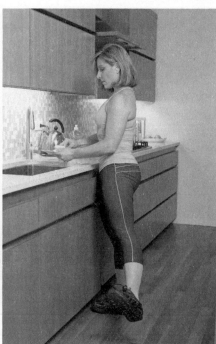

1. Stand close to your sink with your hips resting against it for support and balance.

2. Extend your left leg out to the side, making sure that your tush stays tucked in under you. Flex your foot and bring your leg up about 2–3 inches off the ground, really squeezing your tush. Return your leg to the floor. Flexing your foot helps trim down your saddlebags.

3. Do this for 15–20 reps. NOTE: Place your rinsed dishes on the countertop before loading them into the dishwasher. This will allow you to finish your set without straining your back loading the dishes.

4. With the same leg, foot still flexed, do another 15–20 pulses double time. Really squeeze your tush. Switch legs and repeat.

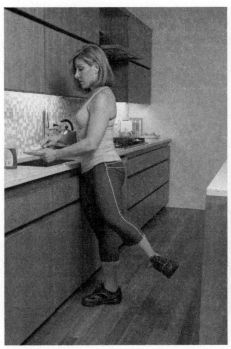 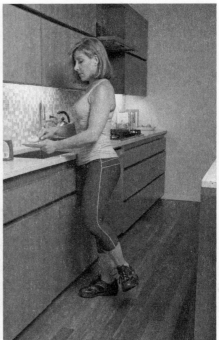

VARIATION:

Face your hips forward and square to the sink, extending your left leg behind you with your knee slightly bent and out to the side. Lift your leg up and down, raising it 2–3 inches off the floor. Do 15–20 reps and really squeeze those glutes! You can also follow the set with 15–20 quick pulses.

Switch legs and repeat, even if your dishes are done. It's only an extra few minutes of your time, and you'll end up with a fab tush!

NOTE: Your foot should never completely touch the ground.

TASKERCISE 5: LIGHTEN YOUR LOAD

WHAT YOU NEED: A dishwasher filled with clean dishes/pots/pans/silverware that needs to be unloaded

WHERE TO DO IT: Kitchen

WHAT IT WORKS: Core, butt, thighs, legs

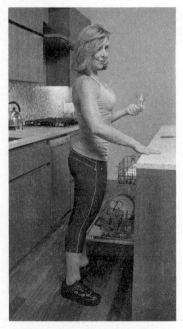 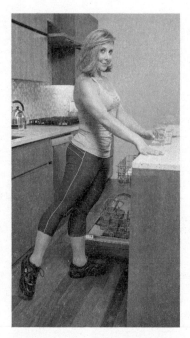 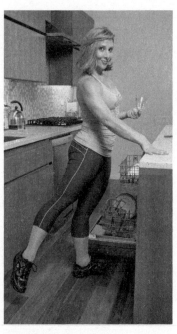

1. Stand to the side or in front of your dishwasher with your feet shoulder-width apart and your toes turned out.

2. Extend your left leg behind you with your toes pointed. As you lift your leg off the ground 2–3 inches, really squeeze your tush, keep your abs tight and your hips square. Reach your leg as far as you can toward the wall behind you, imagining it getting longer. Make sure your foot doesn't touch the ground as you move your leg up and down.

3. Do 15–20 reps with your left leg. Then switch and do the same with your right leg.

TASKERCISE 6: THE DEMI DISH

WHAT YOU NEED: Dishwasher and dishes ready to be loaded

WHERE TO DO IT: Kitchen

WHAT IT WORKS: Core, tush, legs, thighs

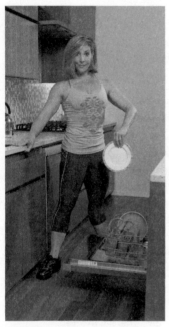 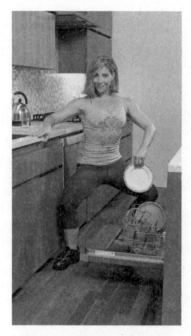 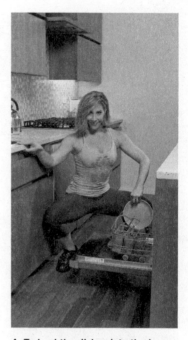

1. Stand to the side or in front of your dishwasher with your feet wide and toes turned out.

2. Bend your knees, making sure your knees don't go past your toes and your tush stays tucked in under you. (This is called a plié in ballet.) Return to starting position and do one set of 15–20 reps.

3. As you plié up and down, really squeeze your thighs and tush on the way up. Over the course of the set, load your rinsed dishes into the dishwasher.

4. To load the dishes into the lower rack, you're going to do the Deep Dish or a grand plié. Bend your knees and follow the instructions above, but this time go deeper toward the floor, allowing your heels to come up.

TASKERCISE 7: CUPBOARD CALF RAISE

WHAT YOU NEED: Cups/glasses that are clean and ready to be stored in cupboards

WHERE TO DO IT: Kitchen

WHAT IT WORKS: Core, tush, and calves

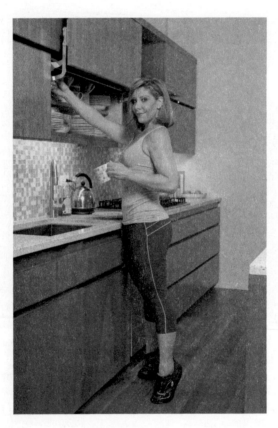

1. Stand facing your cupboard, ready to put away your mugs or glasses two at a time.

2. Balancing carefully (you don't want to drop and break anything!), rise up onto the balls of your feet 5 times while you put your glasses away. Focus on keeping your core strong and your tush tucked in; this will help your balance as well. If the cupboard is high, reach strong and elongate your arms to incorporate some upper-body toning as well.

3. Do 7 Calf Raises while you put away the first two cups; then grab another two. This time do 6 Calf Raises, and grab another two cups. Keep reducing the number of raises until you have worked your way down to 1.

TASKERCISE 8: UNDER THE KNIFE

WHAT YOU NEED: A dishwasher full of clean silverware, waiting to be put away in the drawer

WHERE TO DO IT: Kitchen

WHAT IT WORKS: Core, tush, and thighs

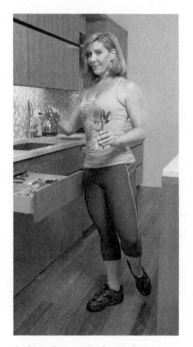 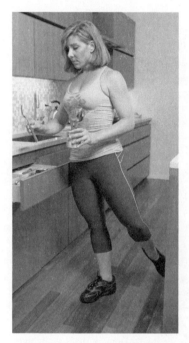 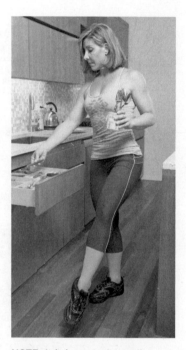

1. Standing tall in front of the silverware drawer with your spine straight, hold your silverware in a cup or tumbler with one hand. You will use your other hand to put away your forks, knives, and spoons.

2. Pull up on your right leg, extending your left leg behind you. Slightly turn your knee out and point your toes.

3. Bring your left leg up 2–3 inches from the floor; then bring it down. Do 15–20 reps as you put your silverware away. Then switch legs.

NOTE: It is important to pull yourself up on your standing leg and not put too much of your weight on it. This will really help with keeping balance, and you'll be working your core muscles as well!

TASKERCISE 9: THE BROOM VROOM

WHAT YOU NEED: Broom, Swiffer, or mop handle

WHERE TO DO IT: Any place that needs sweeping up!

WHAT IT WORKS: Core, thighs, and tush

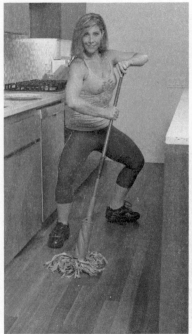 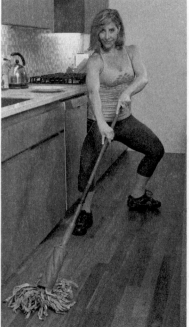 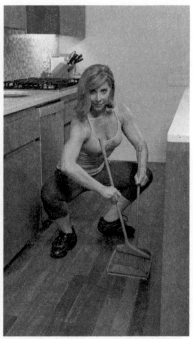

1. Get into a plié position; bending your knees, make sure your knees don't go past your toes. Keep your tush tucked in.

2. As you sweep around you, contract your abs by keeping them really tight.

3. As you go from each section of your floor, get back into your plié position, and make sure that your hips stay still.

VARIATION: DUSTPAN DIPS

1. Stand with your feet shoulder-width apart and your toes turned out. With one hand, hold on to your broom, or duster, and the other hand your dustpan.

2. Make sure your back is straight and your abs are tight as you deeply plié toward the floor.

3. Hold your deep plié position as you sweep your little pile of dirt into the dustpan.

4. To kick it up a notch, pulse for 10 counts as you sweep into your pan.

TASKERCISE 10: STICK IT TO ME

WHAT YOU NEED: Broom, Swiffer, or mop handle

WHERE TO DO IT: Any place that needs sweeping up!

WHAT IT WORKS: Core, thighs, tush, and abs

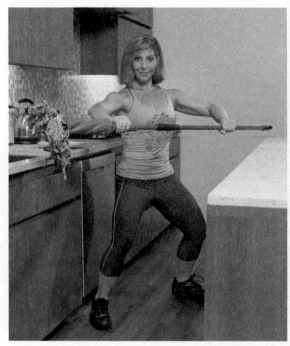 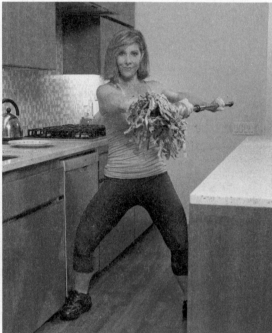

1. Stand up straight and tall with your feet shoulder-width apart, keeping your shoulders down and your abs tight.

2. Hold your broom or your Swiffer with the stick horizontal and your arms straight out in front of you.

3. Get into a deep squat, tucking your tush under you, almost rounding the bottom of your spine. This will really help with keeping your abs contracted.

4. While you are holding this position and your arms are holding your broom straight out in front horizontally (at boob level), twist from the waist up to the left, then back to center, contracting your abs. Repeat to the left 8 times. Make sure you really tuck your tush in and round your lower back.

5. Come back to center and repeat to the right for a total of 8 times.

6. Do this for 30 seconds and work up to 1 minute.

TASKERCISE 11: WAX ON, WAX OFF

WHAT YOU NEED: A paper towel or cloth for polishing/wiping down counters

WHERE TO DO IT: On countertops, bathroom mirrors, shower doors, windows, or any surface that needs shining

WHAT IT WORKS: The Karate Kid's mentor, Mr. Miyagi, was a genius! This move works your upper body and core, tush and thighs (basically, full body). Wave buh-bye to jiggly Jell-O arms!

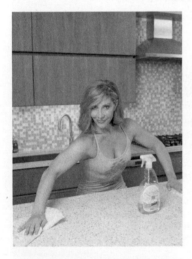
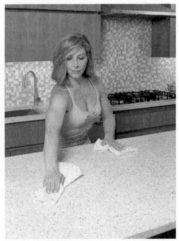

1. Place your legs shoulder-width apart and bend your knees ("plié position" in ballet).

2. Tuck your tush in and engage your abs while standing up tall, with your shoulders down. The more you keep your tummy firm, the more of an ab workout you'll get.

3. Make sure you keep your hips square to the countertop or table you are cleaning.

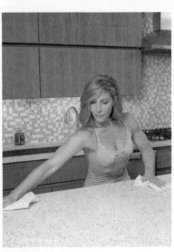
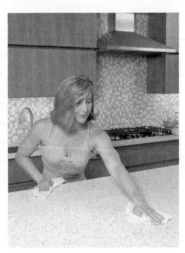

4. Pick an arm to start with. As you clean your countertops, press down hard to create a resistance. Think about isolating the muscles.

5. Do 10 circles on each side, really getting the gunk off your countertops!

6. Do this throughout your day on each countertop.

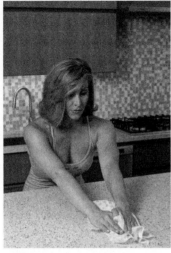
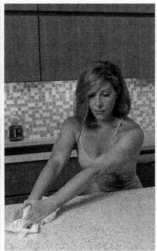
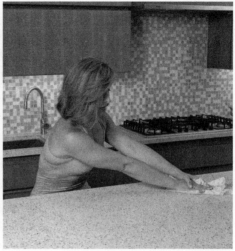

VARIATION 1: WAX ON, WAX OFF, SIDE TO SIDE

1. Start in the same position, standing with your legs shoulder-width apart and your knees bent, tush tucked in, and shoulders down.

2. Place both hands on your towel in front of you.

3. Keeping your abs engaged, wipe your counters from side to side, making sure you are only moving from the waist up. Your hips should stay square to the counter you are working on! No wiggling.

4. Go side to side 10 times, really pushing down on your surface, creating resistance.

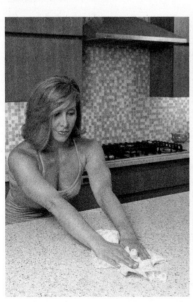
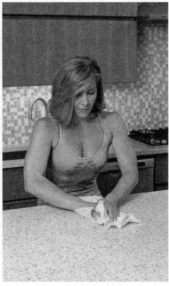

VARIATION 2: WAX ON, WAX OFF, BACK AND FORTH

1. Again, start in the same position, with your legs shoulder-width apart and your knees bent (this will work your quads and tush and is great for your core).

2. Put both hands on your towel and, instead of going side to side, wipe forward and back. As you push out, extend your hands about a foot in front of you, and when you bring your towel back toward your body, push down, creating resistance.

3. Make sure you are using your lower abs to bring your towel back in instead of your arms. Think of your belly button reaching back to your spine.

TASKERCISE 12: THE VACUUM LUNGE

WHAT YOU NEED: A vacuum (either upright or canister with hose attachment)

WHERE TO DO IT: It's my fave anywhere exercise. I don't just do these when I vacuum; I lunge whenever I'm walking around my home, putting things away. But the upright vacuum does help you keep your balance and offers support so you can go low, low, low.

WHAT IT WORKS: All the muscles in your lower body: abs, butt, thighs, calves

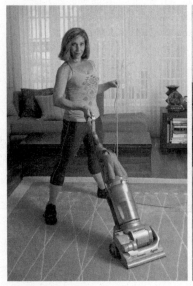
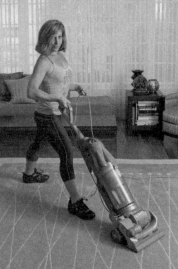
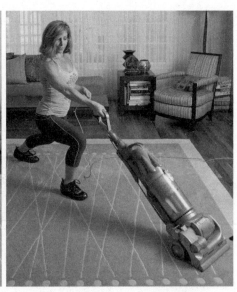

1. Stand behind your vacuum, placing your right hand on the handle.

2. As you begin to vacuum, extend your vacuum out in front of you, stepping forward with your right leg and bending your knee into a lunge. Make sure your knee doesn't go past your toes and stays at a ninety-degree angle.

3. As you vacuum one section of the floor, hold the lunge position, gently pulsing up and down while you move the vacuum back and forth.

4. When it's time to move to a new section of the floor, switch legs and lunge with your left leg. Really engage your abs as you bring your vacuum back and forth.

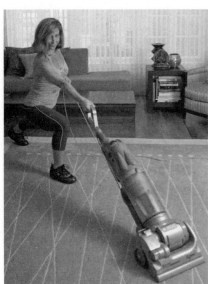 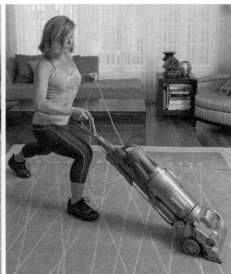

TO REV IT UP:

After you're done vacuuming one room, take a minute to rev it up before you move on to the next room. Get into lunge position and pulse for 30 seconds. The key to pulsing in the lunge is getting low and deep toward the floor but keeping your torso straight and upward. Don't straighten your legs entirely, just stay low with your abs tight. Then switch legs and pulse on the other side. You may have trouble walking the next day, but you'll be one step closer to getting a tight tush!

TASKERCISE 13: SUCK 'N' SQUAT

WHAT YOU NEED: A vacuum (either upright or canister with hose attachment)

WHERE TO DO IT: Living room, bedroom, any room that needs vacuuming (you can do it on hard floors but carpeting offers more resistance)

WHAT IT WORKS: All the muscles in your lower body: abs, butt, thighs, calves

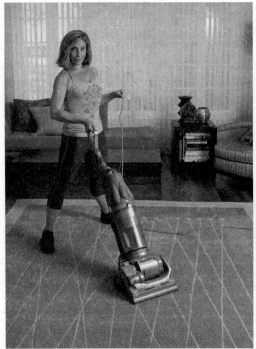 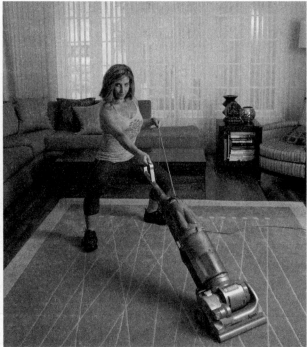

1. Face your vacuum with your feet facing outward at a forty-five-degree angle and shoulder-width apart.

2. Place your right hand on the vacuum.

3. Bend your knees, keeping most of your weight on your heels (make sure your knees don't go beyond your toes).

4. As you extend your arm to vacuum, engage your core and squat down. Don't forget to move your vacuum around your carpet: you don't want to clean just one section.

5. As you stand up, bring your vacuum back toward you. The key to this is to really allow your tummy muscles to do much of the work as you move your vacuum back and forth.

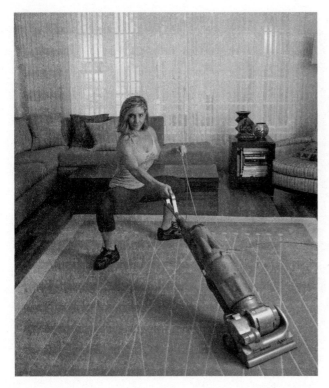

TO REV IT UP: Do 10 Suck 'n' Squats, then hold the squat and pulse for another count of 10.

VARIATION: DEEP SUCK 'N' SQUAT

1. Stand facing your vacuum with your feet shoulder-width apart.

2. This time, instead of having your feet at a forty-five-degree angle, turn them farther outward.

3. As you extend your vacuum out, bend your knees and get really low (don't let your knees go past your toes).

4. Make sure you keep your spine straight, tummy tight, and your tush tucked in.

TO REV IT UP: Do 10 reps, followed by 10 quick pulses at the bottom of your squat, followed by another 10 reps. Your tush will thank you for it!

TASKERCISE 14: SUCK 'N' STRETCH

WHAT YOU NEED: A vacuum (either upright or canister with hose attachment)

WHERE TO DO IT: Living room, bedroom, any room that needs vacuuming (You can do it on hard floors but carpeting offers more resistance.)

WHAT IT WORKS: Arms and abs

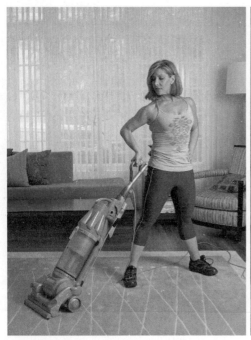 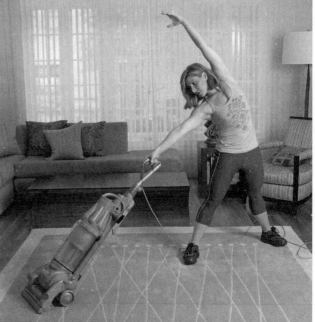

1. Stand with your feet shoulder-width apart and your vacuum on the right side of your right hip.

2. Place your right hand on your vacuum.

3. As you extend your vacuum out to clean, bring your left arm up and over your head and stretch out the left side of your torso.

4. As you bring your vacuum back toward you, bring your left arm back down to your side.

5. Make sure your tush is tucked in, your tummy's tight, and your spine is straight as you bend to the side. The key to this is to keep your body in alignment.

6. Do 10 reps on the left side, then switch to the right.

TO REV IT UP: Combine your Suck 'n' Squat with your Suck 'n' Stretch!

TASKERCISE 15: PILLOW PLUMP AND PUMP

WHAT YOU NEED: Pillows

WHERE TO DO IT: In the bedroom, living room, den . . . anywhere you have pillows that need fluffing

WHAT IT WORKS: This is a good cardio Taskercise that pumps up your heart rate.

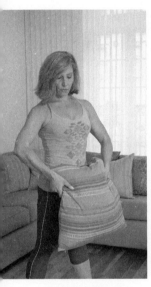 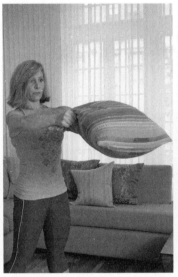 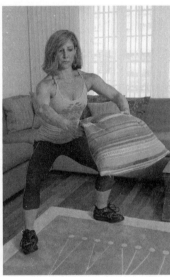 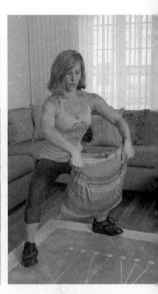

1. Stand with an unfluffed pillow in front of you, one hand on either side of the pillow. Your feet should be shoulder-width apart, with your spine straight, abs tight, and tush tucked in.

2. As you bring your pillow up to fluff it in front of you, fully extend your arms, squeezing your shoulder blades together.

3. The pillow will drop naturally due to gravity. Allow your arms to follow and drop down to your sides. Squat.

4. Repeat 5 times per pillow, squeezing your shoulder blades and your tush.

LAUNDRY

TASKERCISE 16: DETERGENT BOTTLE DUMBBELLS

WHAT YOU NEED: Two full detergent bottles (if they're empty, fill with water); they should weigh about 2 pounds each.

WHERE TO DO IT: Your laundry room or anywhere you store your detergent

WHAT IT WORKS: Shoulders, biceps, back, triceps

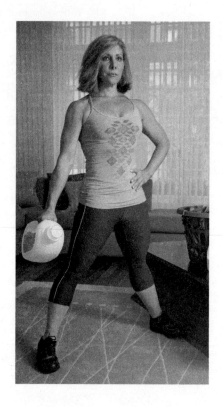

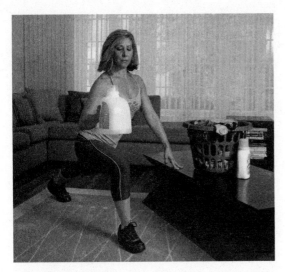 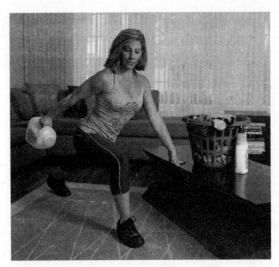

1. Start by holding your detergent bottle with your right hand.

2. Engage your tummy, keep your shoulders down, and straighten your spine.

3. Get into a lunge position, leaning forward with your right leg.

4. Put your other hand on a nearby table, counter, or dryer for support.

5. With your right elbow close to your body, kick back your detergent bottle, squeezing your tricep (aka the back, flabby part of your arm) close to your body as you more your arm backward.

6. As you extend your arm back, straightening it, make sure the upper part of your arm doesn't move.

7. Slowly lower the bottle, then repeat 8–10 times.

8. Switch arms, and switch your front leg, and do 8–10 reps on the other side.

TO REV IT UP: Do 8 reps, then keep your arm kicked back and pulse for another count of 8 before switching arms.

VARIATION 1: DOUBLE KICK-BACK

1. Take one full detergent bottle in each hand, letting your arms hang at your sides. Plant your feet on the floor shoulder-width apart.

2. Leaning forward slightly for balance, extend both arms directly behind you. Hold for a count of 10. Be sure to keep your tummy tight. Think of bringing your belly button closer to your spine.

3. Bring the bottles back toward your hips by bending your elbows and keeping them tight at your sides. Do 8 reps.

VARIATION 2: BOTTLE SALUTE (FOR TRICEPS)

1. Sit with your best posture in a chair. Grab a detergent bottle clasping both hands on the handle.

2. Your elbows should point to the ceiling. Using your elbows as hinges, lift your arms straight up and then lower the detergent bottle back down.

3. Repeat 8 times.

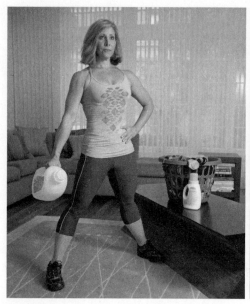
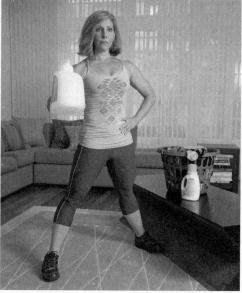

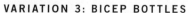

VARIATION 3: BICEP BOTTLES

1. Stand up tall with your tummy engaged and your shoulders down.

2. Take your detergent bottle in your right hand to start.

3. Have your right hand hold the bottle down by your side with your elbow close to your body.

4. You can either rest your left hand on your washing machine for support or place it on your hip.

5. As you inhale, slowly raise your right hand up toward your chest, bringing your elbow to a 90-degree angle.

6. As you exhale, slowly bring your bottle back down. Make sure to maintain control. Don't just drop your arm.

7. Do this exercise slowly, 8 times on each arm.

8. The key to this exercise is to make sure your spine stays straight the entire time; don't lean to the side or let your shoulders climb up to your ears.

TO REV IT UP: Hold one bottle in each hand and alternate arms. Do 16 reps.

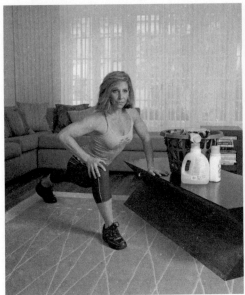

VARIATION 4: LOOSEN-UP LUNGE

1. Lunge forward with your right leg, bending your knee but not extending it beyond your toes.

2. Keep your chest up and sink into the lunge, really stretching out your hip flexor. Hold for 15 seconds.

3. Straighten your right leg and bend forward at the hip, lowering your head over the right leg. Breathe into this stretch, which works your right hamstring.

TASKERCISE 17: BASKET BOOB SQUAT 'N' SQUEEZE

WHAT YOU NEED: Laundry basket of dirty clothes as an added weight before you load your washing machine

WHERE TO DO IT: Your laundry room—or anywhere you are carrying a laundry basket

WHAT IT WORKS: Thighs, tush, core, shoulders, and pecs. This Taskercise will give you perky boobs and a well-lifted tush.

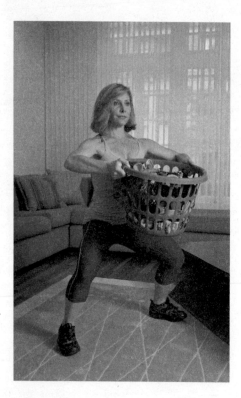

1. Stand with your feet shoulder-width apart and your toes pointing forward.

2. Hold the laundry basket in front of your body with straight arms and one hand on either side of the basket.

3. As you squat down, bring the basket up to boob level with your elbows pointing away from your body. Make sure your shoulders are down even though your elbows are up.

4. Pulse in a squat position for 5 counts, keeping your tush tucked in, your tummy tight, and your shoulders down.

5. As you pulse, squeeze the sides of the basket inward for 5 pulses, working your chest muscles and the inner, flabby part of your arms.

6. Between sets of 5 pulses, come up from your squat. Repeat 2 more times, doing a total of 3 squats and 15 pulses.

TASKERCISE 18: THE LAUNDRY LEG LIFT

WHAT YOU NEED: Laundry in the dryer

WHERE TO DO IT: Anywhere you like to fold your clean wash—a table, a bed, a sofa. All you need is a flat surface.

WHAT IT WORKS: Butt, quads, legs, and core

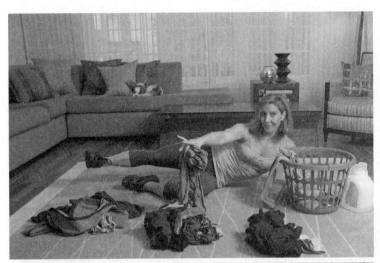

1. Lie on your left side on the floor in front of the laundry that you need to sort. Bend your left leg and extend your right leg with foot flexed.

2. Your left forearm should be bent with the elbow directly under your shoulder for support. Rest your right arm on your right hip. Your hips and shoulders should be stacked up and aligned vertically to the floor. Your head should be aligned with your spine. Engage your tummy muscles to support your spine.

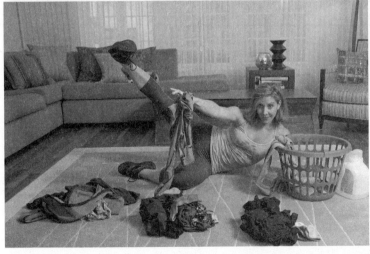

3. Raise your right leg 5–7 inches above your left leg. Keep your hips stacked and aligned to the floor; do not allow them to roll forward or back.

4. Return the right leg to its starting position, moving slowly to maintain full control. Do 3 sets of 15 reps, and then repeat with the left leg.

TASKERCISE 19: TUG-OF-WAR TOWEL TRICEPS

WHAT YOU NEED: A towel, fresh out of the dryer!

WHERE TO DO IT: On the floor, anywhere you like to fold your clean wash

WHAT IT WORKS: Triceps (the back, flabby part of your arms), core, back, and boobs (pectoral muscles)

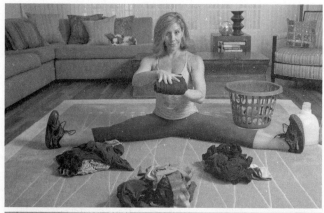

1. Sit on the floor with your legs in a wide V. This helps stretch your hamstrings. Remember to sit tall and keep shoulders down and abs tight.

2. Grab a freshly laundered towel with a hand holding each end.

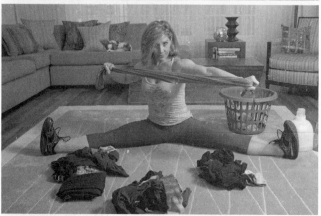

3. Bend your left elbow first, and fully extend your right arm. Hold this position while you pull the towel with both hands.

4. Pull your hands away from each other and do 10 tug-of-war pulses.

5. Switch sides by bending the right elbow an repeat for another 10 times. Try to get in 2–3 sets of 10 on each side.

NOTE: This is a very subtle move, but the harder you tug your with your hands, creating resistance with the towel, the more you will work the muscles. Keep the focus on the triceps, while squeezing your back muscles together.

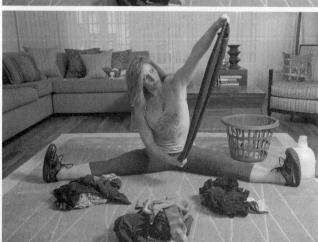

TASKERCISE 20: LAUNDRY BASKET DEEP DIP

WHAT YOU NEED: A laundry basket

WHERE TO DO IT: Your laundry room—or anywhere you are carrying a laundry basket

WHAT IT WORKS: Core, tush, thighs, legs

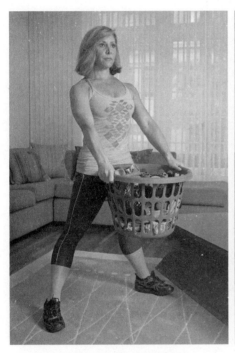 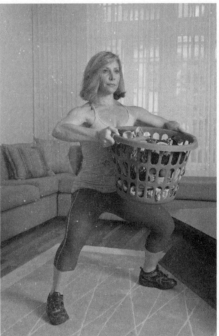

1. Stand with your feet shoulder-width apart, toes slightly turned out. Hold on to your laundry basket with one hand on either side and your arms straight down.

2. Bend your knees and get into a deep dip or plié, making sure your knees don't go beyond your toes, and your tush is tucked in.

3. As you lower into your deep plié, bring your basket up to your waist by bending your elbows.

4. As you straighten your legs to come back up, lower your arms and bring the basket back down. Do 10–12 deep pliés as you bring your laundry basket up and down.

TASKERCISE 21: THE DRESSER DUSTER

WHAT YOU NEED: Dust rag or feather duster, dresser top that needs dusting

WHERE TO DO IT: Bedroom, guest room, kid's room; you can also do this leaning on a wall for support.

WHAT IT WORKS: Core, thighs, legs, tush

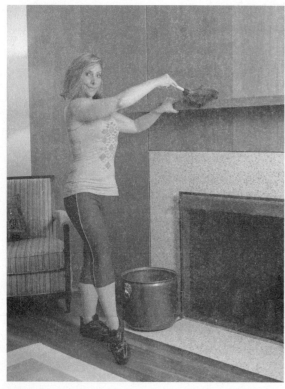 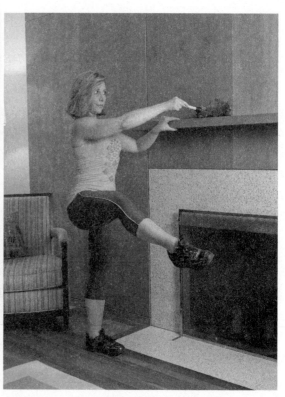

1. Stand to one side of whatever you are dusting, with one hand on the surface for support while the other hand dusts.

2. As you stand tall, with your shoulders down and abs tight, extend your right leg out in front of you and lift it off the ground at least a foot.

3. Bend your knee, turning your leg out so your knee is turned out to the side and not vertical.

4. Lift your leg up and down 10 to 15 times, barely touching your toe to the floor.

TO REV IT UP: Rise up on to your toes as you bring your leg up, and come down on your foot as you bring your leg down, making sure your heel never touches the floor completely.

BATHROOM

TASKERCISE 22: POTTY SQUAT

WHAT YOU NEED: A toilet bowl brush and a potty that needs polishing

WHERE TO DO IT: Bathroom

WHAT IT WORKS: Core, tush, thighs, legs, arms, and abs

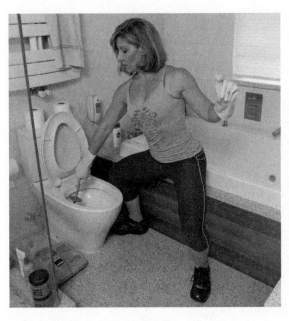

1. Stand facing your toilet, with your feet shoulder-width apart, toes turned out, and with one hand on your toilet brush handle and the other one on your hip.

2. Keeping your body upright (and your nose as far away from the toilet as possible!), squat down into a deep plié. Your back should stay straight; don't hunch over.

3. With the toilet brush, make circles cleaning the toilet bowl, as if you are churning butter. The key here is to keep your abs contracted and steady with non-wiggly hips, so your arms and abs are doing all the work.

DOWN AND DIRTY TIPS: Ring Around the Potty

Alkaline deposits cause those nasty rings! Pour 1 or 2 cups white vinegar into the toilet once a month to eliminate the problem.

A Fresh Bowl Sprinkle ¼ cup baking soda into the toilet bowl. Take your shower and then give the bowl a single scrub. Flush to rinse. Voilà! Instant, odor-free freshness!

TASKERCISE 23: TUB TUSH SQUEEZE

WHAT YOU NEED: A bathtub

WHERE TO DO IT: Bathroom

WHAT IT WORKS: Tush, legs, core, and arms

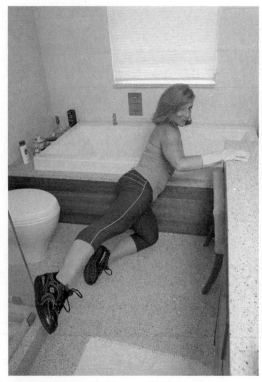 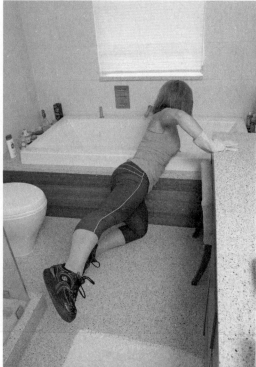

1. Get close to the tub, using one hand to clean and the other for support.

2. As you lean forward to scrub the tub, extend your right leg out straight.

3. Lift your right leg 5–7 inches off the floor while squeezing your tush. It's important to keep your leg completely extended to elongate the muscles.

4. Do 10–15 reps and switch legs.

TASKERCISE 24: TRICEP TUB DIPS

WHAT YOU NEED: A bathtub

WHERE TO DO IT: Your bathroom. This is a great exercise to do while you are giving your kids a bath or waiting for your tub to fill up with water.

WHAT IT WORKS: Jiggly triceps, back, shoulders, core

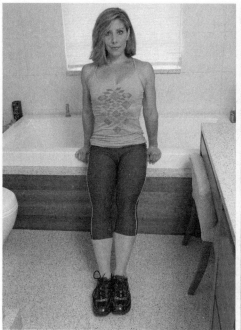 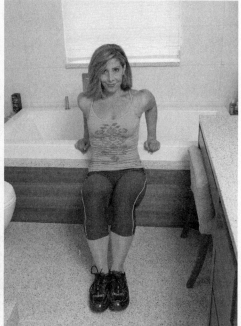

1. Sit up straight and tall, with your shoulders down, on the edge of your tub, facing away from the inside of it.

2. Plant your feet together solidly on the floor.

3. Place your hands on either side of your body with your fingers facing forward.

4. Push your tush off the tub and support yourself with your arms and your core muscles.

5. Bend your elbows as you lower your body toward the ground. Make sure you bend your elbows back and keep them close to your sides. The key to this is to keep your shoulders down, your back straight, and to really make sure your elbows go back and not to the side, so you work your triceps.

6. Get in 10–12 reps. And make sure you stretch afterward. Stand up and clasp your hands behind you. Bend forward with your torso raising your clasped arms up and over your head.

TO REV IT UP: Do an extra 10 mini-pulses after your 10 regular reps.

TASKERCISE 25: **BATHROOM WAX ON, WAX OFF**

WHAT YOU NEED: A towel, cleaner, and a mirror to clean

WHERE TO DO IT: Your bathroom

WHAT IT WORKS: Arms and back

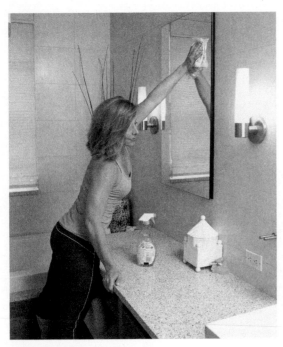
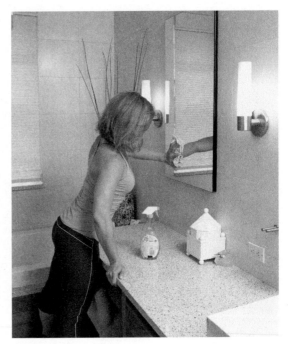

1. Stand facing your mirror with your feet firmly planted on the floor. You may need to rise up onto your toes when you reach up to clean the top of the mirror.

2. After you spray your cleaner on the mirror, make 5 large circles with your left arm as you wipe the mirror. Then make 5 more circles going in the other direction.

3. While you are wiping, be sure not to move from the waist down and to concentrate on isolating the muscles in your core. Remember, the more you push your hand against the mirror, the more resistance you will create and the better your workout will be.

4. Switch to your right arm and repeat 5 large circles in each direction.

cLEAN Momma Boot Camp!

Now that you have the basic Taskercise moves down, it's time to ramp up your workout. You don't need an hour at a gym to get an intense boot-camp workout. All you need is a good thirty-five to forty minutes of elbow-grease cLEANing!

Just Taskercising is great when you are doing your day-in, day-out tasks, like dishes or folding the laundry. The boot camp is for when it's time to really scrub, cLEAN, and sweat! Take the Taskercising exercises I've shown you and mix in some cardio.

THE WARM-UP/PICK-UP

The goal of this warm-up is to get your muscles loose and ready to work. It's also to clear off the countertops, tables, and floors so you can then clean the surface. (You can jump to Wax On, Wax Off on page 116 after you finish!)

If your home has random stuff nesting on your countertops, on the floor, or under the couch, spend three to five minutes walking around your house, taking inventory, and collecting things that need to be put away. Walk at a fast pace while you elevate your heart rate. In order to keep your heart rate up, don't get detail-oriented. What I mean by this is, don't take the time to put your kids' socks in the appropriate drawers: that will slow you down. Instead, put them in the appropriate rooms. Later, when you are working in that room, you can put them away before cleaning the room. Stretch, reach, bend—this will get your body all ready to go for it!

It's also important to stretch before you go for it.

DOWN AND DIRTY TIP: Stain-Busting Baking Soda

Use Arm & Hammer baking soda to remove stains. I make a paste out of baking soda and water, apply it to the stain, and let it sit for an hour before washing the item in the machine. It's amazing how the baking soda zaps the stain away!

BEGINNING YOUR BOOT CAMP

Every person is going to do things differently. You're not going to be able to vacuum, clean your windows, mop the floors, do the laundry, and scrub the toilet in forty minutes or less. So, be practical. If your floors and carpet are gross, choose to only focus on cleaning your floors. If your windows and mirrors need attention, do those. Rotate what needs to get cleaned during the week.

Once you have chosen the rooms or areas of your home that need attention and elbow grease, then you can kick it up a notch. You want to raise your heart rate between Taskercises, and to do this, you'll need to do one of my cardio exercises for at least thirty seconds, pushing your body to the max. What does that mean?

Let's say you are about to clean your tub. Before you do your Taskercises while cleaning your bathtub, do the Football Player for thirty to sixty seconds. Do this as fast and as hard as you can. Note: if you haven't exercised in a while, start out with ten seconds and work your way up. After you have elevated your heart rate, it's time to cLEAN and strengthen. Get in your reps of Tub Tush Squeezes while you clean your tub. Then, as you rinse the residue off, get in your Tricep Tub Dips while the water clears away the gunk. When you are done with your reps, wipe your tub down and move on to the sink.

Before you tackle the built-up toothpaste your kids smeared everywhere, do your cardio blast again, this time choosing jumping jacks. After your heart rate is elevated, slow yourself down and do your Wax On, Wax Off, cleaning your sink and countertop in the bathroom. You get the picture . . . No matter what chore or what room you are

---

DOWN AND DIRTY TIP: A Spotless Shower

If you apply car wax twice a year to the glass doors and walls of your shower (not the floor—it will get slippery!), it will make cleaning easier and keep shiny surfaces from spotting up.

tackling, you are going to mix it up between short bursts of intense cardio and your Taskercises. Use a stopwatch or a clock to keep you on track.

Listen to your body. If you experience pain with any of the exercises, stop and consult your doctor.

Remember:

1. *Go slow!* Listen to your body and know yourself. Don't mistake that for a free pass to not do the work. The only way to really lose weight and see results is to sweat and elevate your heart rate. You will need to build a cardiovascular base if you don't have one. This means starting at a lower intensity and not performing intervals. As you become better conditioned, you will be able to increase your intensity.

2. You can measure your heart rate with a monitor or, as you become more in touch with your body, use what is referred to as RPE (rate of perceived exertion). This is your perception of how hard you are working.

3. You should do short bursts of high-intensity activity followed by a period of active rest (interval training) to make your workout more effective for fat-burning. I suggest doing this type of exercise three times a week: interval training on Monday, Wednesday, and Friday, and walking on Tuesday, Thursday, and Saturday.

CARDIO

CARDIO 1: STAIRCASE

If you have a set of stairs . . . *score!* Use them!

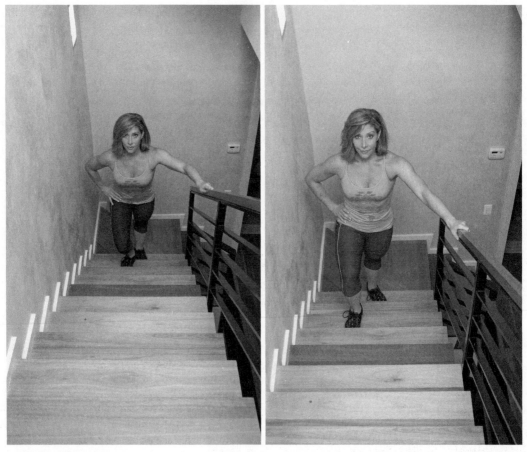

1. If you are already going upstairs, take 30–60 seconds and go as quickly and as many times as you can up and down your stairs.

2. Remember, you can hold on lightly to your railing to keep your balance, but don't use it as a crutch. Keep your spine straight and your tummy tight as you push yourself to the max, bringing your heart rate up, as well as toning your tush!

CARDIO 2: STAIR EXERCISES

After you increase your heart rate by going up and down the stairs for 30–60 seconds at your body's full capacity, work your tush, thighs, and core by doing these additional stair exercises.

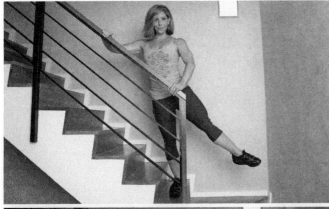

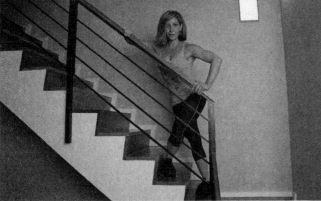

1. Start at the bottom of the stairs facing the banister, gently placing your hands on it for support. Extend your left leg out to your side, pointing your toes.

2. Step up one stair with your left foot. Raise your right foot from the lower step and place it next to your left. Now extend your left leg out to the side and point your toes. Make sure your abs are tight and your body is pulled up and square to the banister. Don't raise your hips. Really squeeze your tush!

3. Cross your left leg in front of your right foot and step up onto the next step.

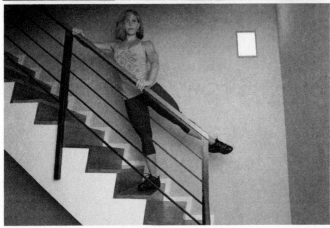

4. After you place your left foot down on the next step, raise your right foot from the lower step and place it next to the left. Extend your left leg to the side again.

5. Continue climbing the stairs, extending the left leg each time you ascend to a higher step.

6. When you get to the top of the stairs, quickly go back down to the bottom and repeat steps 1–5 with your right leg.

CARDIO 3: THE FOOTBALL PLAYER

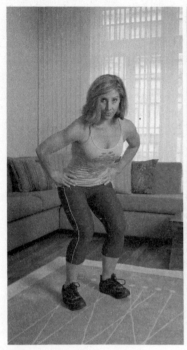 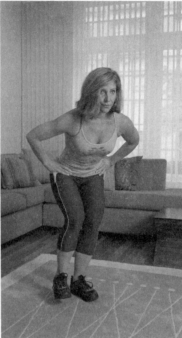 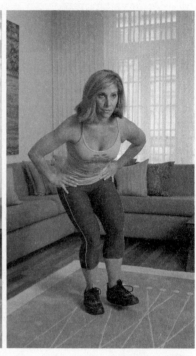

1. Stand with your feet together, engaging your tummy muscles, and bend your knees. Run in place but never actually lift your feet off the ground. With your weight mostly on your heels, stay flat on your foot as you alternate feet, as fast as you can, for 30–60 seconds.

2. The lower and deeper you get, the more you'll feel the burn!

3. Remember to breathe. Inhale deeply through your nose, exhale through your mouth. Don't slow down; push yourself!

CARDIO 4: IMAGINARY JUMP ROPE

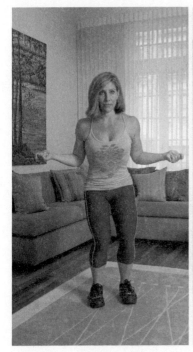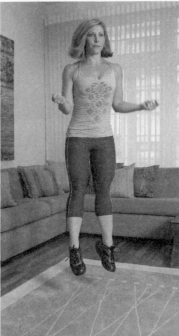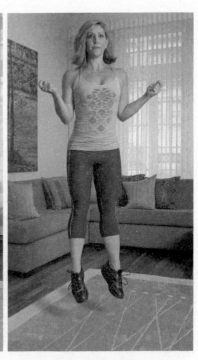

1. Stand up straight and tall, engaging your core.

2. Pretend you are holding a jump rope. Keep your elbows close to your sides.

3. As you rotate your imaginary jump rope around your body, keep your elbows tight to your body and jump twice per rotation. Do this for 30–60 seconds, pushing your body to its full capacity if you can.

4. Be sure that when you land, you come down on your toes and then your heels in order to absorb the shock on your knees. Bend your knees deeply before jumping again.

CARDIO 5: JUMPING JACKS

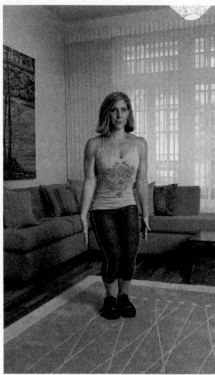 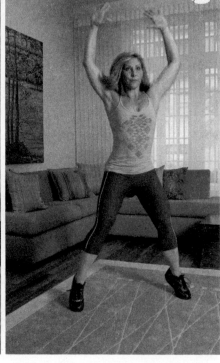

1. Start in a standing position with your feet together and your arms by your sides.

2. Bend your knees.

3. Jump so that your feet are shoulder-width apart.

4. While jumping, raise your arms up above your head.

5. Then jump back from your wide stance and bring your arms back down to your sides. Make sure that your spine is straight and your core is engaged. As you land from your jump, go from toe to heel; this will help protect your knees when you land. The key with jumping jacks is to sustain them for 30–60 seconds. Push your body to its full capacity if you can.

Target Taskercise

Most people have love/hate relationships with their bodies—as in, "I love my arms and hate my thighs." Taskercise is an easy way to target those problem areas. I recommend doing 20–30 minutes of cardio and these groups of exercises.

If you really want to benefit and target those trouble spots, I suggest sneaking Taskercises in three times per day, three to four days a week. To really kick it up a notch, raise your heart rate 1–2 minutes before you do each set. You can refer to my quick and simple "anywhere" cardio bursts (beginning on page 140) for help.

To achieve . . .

FAB ABS:

> Playtime Crunch (see page 187)
>
> Snow Angels (see page 187)
>
> Taskercise 11: Wax On, Wax Off (variation, Side to Side)
>
> Taskercise 2: The Rag Drag Twist

TONED ARMS/PERKY BOOBS:

> Taskercise 3: Time Press
>
> Taskercise 16: Detergent Bottle Dumbbells (variation, Double Kick Back)
>
> Taskercise 17: Basket Boob Squat 'n' Squeeze
>
> Taskercise 24: Tricep Tub Dips

(continued)

TIGHT TUSH:

> Taskercise 12: The Vacuum Lunge
>
> Taskercise 13: Suck 'n' Squat, Deep Suck 'n' Squat
>
> Taskercise 23: Tub Tush Squeeze
>
> Taskercise 4: Suds Me Up!
>
> The Hotel Wall Squat (see page 178)

SEXY LEGS:

> Taskercise 19: The Laundry Leg Lift (to the back and side)
>
> Taskercise 23: Tub Tush Squeeze
>
> Taskercise 21: The Dresser Duster
>
> Taskercise 4: Suds Me Up!

CHART: Taskercise Log

When you keep this Taskercise log, you will see just how much you've worked out—and how much you've accomplished.

CHART 1: CARDIO

	SET ONE TIME/ QUANTITY	SET TWO TIME/ QUANTITY	SET THREE TIME/ QUANTITY	SET FOUR TIME/ QUANTITY
CLEAN MOMMA RAG DRAG				
JUMPING JACKS				
MARCHING IN PLACE				
OTHER				

Suggested time: 10–15 minutes throughout workout or do 2–3 sets of 10–15 reps per exercise.

CHART 2: STRENGTH

	SET ONE TIME/ QUANTITY	SET TWO TIME/ QUANTITY	SET THREE TIME/ QUANTITY	SET FOUR TIME/ QUANTITY
WAX ON, WAX OFF CIRCLES				
WAX ON, WAX OFF SIDE TO SIDE				
TIME PRESSES				
SUDS ME UP				
COOL-DOWN STRETCHES				
OTHER				

Suggested time: 10–15 minutes throughout workout or do 2–3 sets of 10–15 reps per exercise.

Cool-Down Stretches

I try to stretch after every time I do a set of Taskercises. And twice when I do my boot camp (before and after). Here are my top favorites that take only a sec to do wherever, whenever!

TAKE A BOW STRETCH

This is amazing to do after you sneak in your Time Presses, if you've been sitting at a computer for a while, or whenever you're feeling tight in your shoulders and neck.

1. Stand with your feet shoulder-width apart, shoulders down.

2. Clasp your hands behind your back and really feel the stretch in your chest.

3. Bow your head and bend your body forward, one vertebra at a time, keeping your hands clasped together.

4. Reach your clasped hands over your head, or as best you can. Let your head drop completely.

5. Inhale through your nose and out through your mouth several times.

6. Slowly come up one vertebra at a time.

SINK PULL DOWN

This works the sides of your torso, your arms, your lower back, and your hamstrings, all of which contribute to lower-back pain when tight. (See the right photo on page 107 for an example.)

1. Stand with your feet shoulder-width apart and about two feet away from your sink.

2. Extend your arms out and grab on to your sink.

3. As you lean back and into a stretch, continue to hold on to the sink.

4. Drop your head and relax your shoulders. Do not lock your knees as you hold this position.

5. Curl the lower part of your back by tucking your tush in.

6. Take five deep inhales through your nose, exhaling through your mouth.

FAB "4" STRETCH

This works your lower back and glutes. It's great after cardio or a leg-lift series. It's also a great exercise for relieving lower-back pain and sciatica.

1. Stand sideways, with your hip next to a counter or a sturdy chair and your feet together. Hold on to the counter or chair back for support.

2. Take your outside leg (the leg that is farthest from the counter or chair) and place your ankle over the knee of the opposite leg. It should look like you have made the number 4.

3. With your knees turned out, sit into this position, really stretching out those glutes.

4. Inhale through your nose, and exhale through your mouth 5 times on each side.

SMELL MY PITS STRETCH

This is fab for stretching your chest, front shoulders, and abs. You'll need a towel.

1. Sit on the floor in a cross-legged position (or, as my son, Jack, likes to say, "crisscross applesauce").

2. Hold the towel with both hands slightly more than shoulder-width apart, arms extended overhead.

3. Lift your chest and arch your upper back slightly as you pull out gently on the ends of the towel. Make sure you don't arch your lower back too much. Do it 3–5 times while breathing slowly.

You're Never Too Old to Taskercise!

Anyone, and I mean *anyone*, can Taskercise—even my sixty-eight-year-old mother-in-law, Bubbie! Bubbie is a fantabulous combination of George Costanza's mom and Gracie Allen. She loves her grandchildren more than a bowl of matzo ball soup from Brent's Deli, and she's as loving as she is a ding-dong (I mean that in the kindest way!). She always means well, but listening and paying attention to the world around her are not her priority. This is a woman who will eat a box of Jujubes and wonder why her dentures are stuck to the roof of her mouth!

Bubbie swears she exercises daily; however, her idea of exercise is chasing her three crazy dogs down the block every morning while wearing her slippers. Bubbie is always on a diet for a minute and a half. She'll try something new, be so excited, and then spend more time talking about her diet than actually staying on her diet. The long and short of this . . . Ya gotta love Bubbie.

That being said . . . I finally put her straight and cLEANed up her thinking! I said, "Laney, ya gotta come cLEAN with yourself! Seriously! If you want to live a longer, healthier, happier life, you have to make some changes. I know you have problems with your hips, you have chronic pain and osteoporosis. I know you have acid reflux. I know your sleep isn't always the best. But complaining about it and *pretending* to do something about it is as bad, if not worse, than sitting in front of the TV night after night eating your Jujubes." She looked at me as if I had two heads . . . but some of it got through to her.

I find that the older people get, the more set they are in their ways and habits (myself included). Change is a bitch. The key, I told her, is to make it manageable. Don't go jogging if you have trouble with your knees. I gave Bubbie a few Taskercises to help tone up her arms and strengthen her core. I taught her how to incorporate them into her daily life. "This is doable!" she reported back to me. As a result, she lost inches around her hips, thighs, and waist, and her lower-back pain eased up. She also told me that she was sleeping better and not waking up as much in the middle of the night. Seriously, if Bubbie can Taskercise, so can you!

DOWN AND DIRTY TIP: Pet Hair Be Gone!

 You can use a wet rubber dishwashing glove or even a baby wipe to wipe away pet hair. It's so easy and takes only two seconds!

Burn It with Bubbie!

Here's the deal, ladies: the secret to staying young is staying active. Muscle mass decreases as you age. And you need that muscle: it keeps you strong, burns calories, helps you maintain your weight, and contributes to balance and bone strength. Regular exercise can help boost your energy and manage the symptoms of any illness or pain. It can even reverse some of the symptoms of aging. And not only is exercise good for your body—it's also good for your mind, mood, and memory. Regular exercise and core strengthening can help with balance, hypertension, diabetes, arthritis pain, anxiety, and depression.

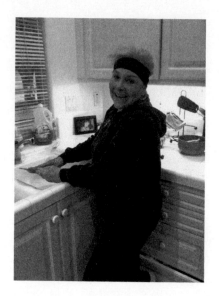

Stay strong, stay fit, stay independent! And don't think it's too late for you if you're in your golden years! You're never too old to exercise! If you've never exercised before, or it's been a while, start with light walking and other gentle activities.

The main exercises seniors should focus on are:

- **Endurance activities, such as walking for twenty minutes a day. These build staying power and will improve your overall health, your heart, and your circulatory system.**

- **Strengthening exercises, such as Soup-Can Shoulder Lifts on page 153. These will build muscle tissue and reduce age-related muscle loss.**

- **Stretching exercises, such as the Wall-to-Wall Stretch below. These help keep your body limber and flexible.**

- **Balancing exercises, such as Heel-Toe Stroll on page 155. These will help reduce your chances of falling.**

BUBBIE-CISE 1: WALL-TO-WALL STRETCH

You can do this one during a commercial break—a good thing, since Bubbie wouldn't want to miss a minute of *Magnum PI*. (Tom Selleck is "to die for.") This exercise increases the flexibility of your arms, chest, and shoulders. Stretching out those areas in your body will make it easier for you to reach things on high shelves, like in your closet or kitchen cabinets.

1. Stand facing a wall, slightly farther than an arm's length from it, feet shoulder-width apart.

2. Lean your body forward and put your palms flat against the wall at shoulder height and shoulder-width apart.

3. Keeping your back straight, slowly walk your hands up the wall until your arms are above your head.

4. Hold your arms overhead for 10–30 seconds.

5. Slowly walk your hands back down to shoulder height.

6. Repeat at least 3–5 times.

BUBBIE-CISE 2: SOUP-CAN SHOULDER LIFT

Use your canned soup, or any other canned food, as an opportunity to strengthen your shoulder and arm muscles (less aches and pains!). Bubbie does this before heating up some soup on the stove, or when putting groceries away.

1. Sit in a chair with your back straight. Keep your feet planted on the floor and shoulder-width apart.

2. Your arms should be straight down at your sides, with your palms facing inward and your hands holding on to your soup cans.

3. Holding your cans in either hand, raise both arms out to the sides at shoulder height. Hold the position for one second.

4. Slowly lower your arms to the sides. Pause. Repeat 8–15 times.

5. Rest. Do another set of 8–15 repetitions.

DOWN AND DIRTY TIP: Baby Oil Isn't Just for Babies!

My sister Deb taught me about the many magical uses of baby oil. If your necklaces get knotted, pour a bit of baby oil over them and untangle with a pin. Another great use is removing Band-Aids from boo-boos. My son would scream every time I tried to peel his bandage off. But if you lather some baby oil on top, it slides right off, with no sticky goo.

BUBBIE-CISE 3: SOUP-CAN BICEP CURLS

This Taskercise is great for strengthening your upper-arm muscles.

1. Sit in your chair, keeping your feet flat on the floor and shoulder-width apart.

2. Hold your soup can with your right hand. Keep your arm straight, with your palm facing toward your body. Your other hand can hold on to the chair for support.

3. Slowly bend your elbow, lifting your soup can toward your chest. Make sure you keep your abs tight and your shoulders down. Hold the position for one second.

4. Slowly lower your arm to the start position.

5. Do it 8–10 times, then repeat with your other arm.

6. Rest. Then do another set of 8–10, alternating arms.

BUBBIE-CISE 4: SIT AND STAND

This exercise will strengthen your core and thigh muscles and will also help with your balance. It's a great one to do when you're watching TV.

1. Place a pillow against the back of your chair.

2. Sit in the middle or toward the front of the chair, knees bent, feet flat on the floor.

3. Lean back on the pillow in a half-reclining position, keeping your back and shoulders straight.

4. Raise your upper body forward until you are sitting upright, using your hands as little as possible, or ideally, not at all. Your back should no longer lean against the pillow.

5. Keeping your tummy muscles tight, slowly stand up, using your hands as little as possible.

6. Now slowly sit back down. Keep your tummy tight and your back and shoulders straight throughout the exercise. The more you are aware of your posture, the better chance you have of improving your balance.

7. Repeat 8–15 times.

8. Rest. Then repeat 8–15 times more.

BUBBIE-CISE 5: HEEL-TOE STROLL

Instead of just walking to the bathroom—or any room, for that matter—go heel-to-toe, to build your balance.

1. Stand up tall and straight.

2. Position the heel of one foot right in front of the toes of the other foot. Your heel and toes should touch or almost touch.

3. Choose a spot ahead of you and focus on it to keep you steady as you walk.

4. Take a step. Put your heel just in front of the toe of your other foot.

5. Repeat for 20 steps.

6. Straighten your arms out to the sides to help your balance.

cLEAN Momma Pop Quiz: What's Your Workout Personality?

If you're going to stick to a workout plan, you need it to be one that works for you. For starters, what kind of an exerciser are you? Evaluate your answers below; then you'll see the best places/times to fit Taskercise into your life.

Exerciser Type 1: The Loner

I like to work out:

- ❏ in my home
- ❏ privately; with no one watching
- ❏ early in the morning or late at night, when the house is quiet

Exerciser Type 2: The Team Player

I like to work out:

- ❏ with my friends
- ❏ while spending time with my kids/hubby
- ❏ in a public place, like a park, surrounded by other people working out. It motivates me!

Exerciser Type 3: The No-Time-to-Waster

I like to work out:

- ❏ whenever I can find a spare minute
- ❏ while doing something else: talking on the phone, making dinner, folding laundry
- ❏ at the office—I'll take the steps over the elevator any day!

Exerciser Type 4: The Easy Does It-er

I like to work out:

- ❏ in air-conditioning. I hate to sweat!
- ❏ in my bedroom, living room, den
- ❏ in whatever is comfy: old T, baggy sweats, bra/panties!

Exercise Type 5: Wherever, Whenever

I like to work out:

- ❑ on vacations—it's no time to slack off!

- ❑ whenever the mood strikes me—even if it's at the grocery store

- ❑ without fancy equipment/machines

DOWN AND DIRTY TIP: Boo-boo Stain Remover

My son, Jack, had a little boo-boo on his finger and got hysterical once he saw blood (mind you, it was a little cuticle cut). Needless to say, he used my cute blue shirt as a tissue, wiping his little bloody finger and his runny nose all over it. *Gross!* Blood stains are tough, but not if you try this trick: make a paste of cool water and meat tenderizer. Apply to the stain, let sit fifteen to thirty minutes, then wash.

cLEAN Routine

7
Clear Out Clutter

cLEAN Momma Says . . . When you keep less stuff lying around, you enjoy life more. It's a case of simplifying, of paring down to what you really need/want/use.

YOUR CHAPTER 7 LAUNDRY LIST

- **Bit by bit, start to let go of the clutter in your home and your life. Tackle one small area at a time.**
- **Learn what you need to live and what you can live without.**
- **Organize your home so you can be more efficient with your time and space.**

I'm gonna come clean here . . . I am no organizing expert. In fact, I am quite challenged in this department. Don't get me wrong: I hate clutter and mess, and my house is very simplified and tidy. That being said, I am incredibly challenged keeping it this way. Piles of crap can easily accumulate into a world of chaos in a matter of minutes! So you will find that most of my tips in this chapter are for the severely organizationally challenged, like myself. I like to make life as easy as possible. So, if you're with me on that point . . .

Why Is It Important to De-clutter?

De-cluttering is ridding your space of anything not useful or necessary. Clutter on the outside is often a reflection of clutter on the inside. The more space you make, the easier it is for you to find things, do things, make your life more efficient. If you're buried under a hunk of junk, nothing is going to get done! A lot of people are afraid to de-clutter (guilty as charged!). There's a sense of loss involved; you have to get *rid* of clutter to make it go away. Many of my clients tell me they worry they'll need the items later . . . or they claim some deep, sentimental attachment to the item. Yeah, I was sentimentally attached to about ten pairs of shoes too many. Get over it! It's an object, not an individual. It won't cry if you give it away. Other people think, "Well, I paid for it . . . so I should keep it." But does it have any value to you now? Are those knickknacks collecting dust on your shelf really serving any purpose—or might you be better off selling them on eBay? That's a way to make some of your money back!

My point is this: you can come up with a million and one excuses why you should stay cluttered. That isn't getting you anywhere—in fact, it's holding you back. And it isn't just material stuff that can pile up: it can be tasks, appointments, projects, even ideas. Your mind can be cluttered as well. I've worked hard to de-clutter my space and my psyche, and I can truthfully say I don't miss anything. I feel more in control and less burdened. Plus, there's a lot less junk to trip over!

The hardest part of de-cluttering is getting started. Where do you begin? What do you toss? What do you keep? Here's my system:

A PLACE FOR EVERYTHING AND EVERYTHING IN ITS PLACE. Start by picking up five things that you actually use (your fave mug's been hanging out on the counter; your hairbrush on the sink; your kids' Nintendo DS on the dining room table) and finding good places for them. Take a minute to think—where would be a good spot? It should be somewhere easily accessible but also tucked away so it looks tidy.

FIND CREATIVE WAYS TO ORGANIZE. I love using Tupperware containers to store everything from my kids' crayons and paints to extension cords and spare tubes of toothpaste. You can also recycle old coffee cans, tissue boxes, and clear jars to sort and store your stuff. Putting things into smaller, organized compartments gives you a sense of visual order.

START WITH FIVE MINUTES A DAY. Set a goal for yourself to tackle one small spot at a time. If you announce, "I'm going to de-clutter my entire house today!" you'll give yourself both a hernia and a nervous breakdown. Pick one place that's maybe been overrun forever: a closet, a desk drawer, the cabinet under your kitchen sink, and work your way through it, bit by bit. You won't make a huge dent, but it's a beginning. If you're motivated, do more. Otherwise, tomorrow is another day!

Go through each space, emptying it out so you can really see what's hiding in there. When you've sorted through, put back the stuff you love and use, neatly. You may want to find better ways to store it. Whatever you're not keeping, place into a box to be donated or recycled or given to friends and family. Better their house than yours!

CHUCK THIS! In general, if something is torn, stained, broken beyond repair . . . out it goes. Was it in style in the '70s? Hasn't fit in five years? Adios, amigo! Expired, exploded (yup, see what happens when you leave a Coke can in the pantry for two years!), unidentifiable (was that makeup . . . or my kid's science project in that bottle?): purge, purge, purge!

OUT WITH THE OLD BEFORE IN WITH THE NEW. Don't buy yourself a new dress, pair of shoes, etc., without getting rid of at least one you no longer need or want. I like to make three piles when I'm going through closets and drawers: keep, toss, maybe. This helps me to do a quick sort and make decisions before I have time to change my mind! Assign a recipient for what you want to get rid of: a charity, a relative who wants hand-me-downs, a local school or nursing home, church/synagogue, Goodwill. When you have a happy home for your items to go to, it's easier to get rid of them.

De-cluttering Room by Room

As I've said before, I'm a problem solver. I like to look at each area in my home as its own unique clutter zone and tackle it differently.

THE BATHROOM

One of the biggest clutter culprits in the loo is what I refer to as "bottle bulk." Have you ever noticed how many products you have in there that are *almost* empty but not quite? I start by going through **MY SHOWER AND THE CABINET UNDER MY SINK**. I first see if there are several bottles containing the same conditioner, shampoo, body wash, etc. If there are, I combine them and toss the empty bottles out for recycling or use them for art projects (my kids love to turn them into flower vases and pencil holders). If there are tiny amounts left of lots of different products, I choose one empty bottle and fill it with them, creating a soapy mixture my kids can use to shampoo their dolls' hair or wash toy cars.

Next comes the **MEDICINE CABINET**. If you don't have one spot for medicines, create one now. Make sure it's out of reach of little fingers (kids can mistake pills or vitamins for candy). Go through everything for the outdated medicines, the creams that did nothing to rid you of wrinkles, your fifty shades of pink lipstick. Simplify to the essentials and get rid of any product past its prime (a three-year-old mascara is a good example!). And always make sure you have the emergency OTC drugs on hand: pain and fever relievers (for adults as well as kids); first-aid supplies (bandages, antibiotic ointment, rubbing alcohol, gauze); allergy meds (e.g., children's Benadryl); cough syrup; and a thermometer. If your child has special medications, such as an inhaler for asthma, make sure that's up to date as well and in plain sight.

I use my **TUPPERWARE CONTAINERS** to keep everything organized, and I label the lids with Sharpies so I know what's inside. I have a Mommy's Headache Box filled with Advil and Tylenol. Maybe I should consider storing a bottle of vodka in there, too? There's a Tummy Box for antacids, Pepto, and Imodium; a Vitamin Box, containing all the alphabet letters (vitamins A, B, C, D, etc.) I take on a regular basis; and a Boo-boo Box filled with tweezers, colorful, cartoony bandages of assorted sizes, antiseptic, etc., so when I have a bleeding, hysterical kid, I have just one place to go to make it all better!

DOWN AND DIRTY TIP: Brush Out the Grass

My kids and I love to roughhouse in our grassy yard. That, of course, means grass stains on my knees and tush! I learned this trick from my sister Deb. Instead of brushing your teeth, brush out the grass! Get an old toothbrush, rub some whitening toothpaste into your stain, and let it sit overnight. Then wash and presto! Bye-bye, grassy butt!

THE BEDROOM

My bedroom is usually the last area I organize, when, in truth, it should be the first! It's the place where I start and finish my day. When my bedroom is cluttered and overflowing with random, unnecessary things, it makes it hard for me to relax. So instead of sleeping and waking surrounded by clutter, I created a sanctuary—my momma cave.

Bedroom Closets

Start with your closets. First, get rid of anything I described in the "Chuck This!" section on page 163 that you will never wear: items that are too soiled, ripped, or ruined. Then search out the stuff you haven't worn in the last six months. If you haven't missed these things in all that time, you're not gonna miss them now. Move on to purging what I call "hopeful" clothes—the size 2 jeans you wore in college, the evening gown you swear will fit if you only lose ten pounds. If you reach your weight-loss goal, buy yourself a new outfit!

Get rid of shoes that are painful, broken, or missing their match. I can guarantee you that the fabulous pair of overpriced heels you impulsively bought online will never be worn (despite the occasion you bought them for) if they kill your feet. Same goes for scarves, hats, and belts that don't coordinate with anything in your closet. (I know, I know . . . you were sure that pink leopard pashmina was going to become the staple of

The Best Way to Organize Your Closet

- **THE SHORT AND THE LONG OF IT.** Group all of the long hanging clothes (coats, dresses) on one side and the short hanging clothes (folded pants, shirts) on the other. You'll create the feeling of more space. And underneath the short stuff, you can use that space, too. I like to store a hamper under there, see-through shoe or sweater boxes, or plastic containers with pull-out drawers.

- **"NO WIRE HANGERS!"** Mommy Dearest was right! Get matching slim, inexpensive hangers and ditch the wire ones from the dry cleaner. They only get mangled and your clothes fall off them easily. If your hangers are all the same size, type, and color, it gives the illusion of a more organized space.

- **COORDINATE BY COLOR.** I found this to be calming, and it makes getting ready and spotting my fave blue tank infinitely easier. If reorganizing into a rainbow is too much for you to handle, then go from darks (black, navy, brown) to lights (white, beige) and brights.

- **SEASONALLY STORE AND STASH.** Take all your bulky sweaters and puffy jackets out of your closet when it's ninety degrees out. You can easily fold them up and stash them in a large box under your bed. I also know people who store all their winter wear at the dry cleaner or in a storage locker. It's a small price to pay for an organized closet!

your wardrobe!) You may have to be a bit merciless in your closet editing, but you'll be grateful when you have more space and can actually see what you own. Which brings me to . . .

Drawers

Sometimes I peer into my sock drawer and all I see is chaos: socks that have holes in them or have no match, striped tights that make my thighs look fat, dozens of pairs of pantyhose that have sprung a run. Take it all out and sort it so you can see what needs to go and what can stay. Then get a drawer organizer. These are fun little plastic boxes or separators that keep your panties apart from your bras, T-shirts, and other items.

This is a huge time-saver that allows you to grab and go (and many a time has saved me the embarrassment of leaving my home panty-less!).

The Nightstand

For many people, this is also known as the "dumping ground." A lovely little spot to toss all your loose stuff at the end of the day. If you have drawers, you have my permission to make one of them the "junk drawer." But the other should be organized and efficient: a place for your earplugs, your book, your medication, a flashlight, your hand cream, some condoms, the things you need as part of your bedtime routine. On top, only have what you use or what makes you feel happy and calm—a pretty candle, a framed photo, a treasured tchotchke. No millions of magazines or newspapers piled to the ceiling (you can only read one at a time!). No tangled earrings, necklaces, and rings you are too lazy to put in your jewelry box.

YOUR HOME OFFICE

A messy desk can be debilitating! It can stop your brain from being creative or from getting tasks done. "Outta sight, outta mind" doesn't work for my health insurance bill that's hiding under my kid's report card.

    TAME THE PAPER PILEUPS. They usually occur because you're never sure what you one day might need . . . so you keep it all. It's just a single sheet of paper, right? Well, those sheets seem to mate and multiply . . . because I find mountains of them all over my home. And half the time, I have no idea what's on them or why I saved them! The solution: find a better way to keep them. File them in a drawer, tuck them into a large manila envelope or accordion folder, clip them or staple them together according to subject, place them in a binder. Go through them every week, so they don't have a chance to grow. Once or twice a week, I spend a few minutes going through all the mini-piles stashed around my kitchen, desk, or nightstand, and file them.

    I also make two piles on my desk. On the left side, I put all my completed documents and important papers that don't need my immediate attention. Then, when I have a moment to spare, I sort and file them. On the right side, I have my "Need to do" pile. This is where I stack the bills that need to be paid, the permission slips that need to be signed, etc. This pile is always neat and easily accessible—so I'll get to it!

THE KITCHEN

Pick the cupboard you want to start with and empty it all out, including cabinet organizers, such as racks and shelf dividers, as well as food, appliances, pots and pans, dishes, cups, mugs. Wipe down the entire space, getting out all the crumbs, dust, and spills. Now put "like things" together on each shelf when you replace them: cups together, glasses together, etc. Toss away anything that's chipped, old, or gross. I keep the stuff that is most frequently used front and center, so it's accessible. For example, I won't keep the pretty crystal cake plate I got as a wedding gift in front of my pots and pans in the cupboard, especially when I don't bake! I have a fairly simple system:

- **SPICES: I keep my spices near my food, work/prep area, and stove. This way, they are easily accessed while I'm prepping, chopping, and mixing.**

- **GLASSES AND DISHES: I put these things in the cabinets right above my dishwasher; that way I can easily put them away when my dishwasher is done cleaning.**

- **POTS AND PANS: I store my pots and pans in a cupboard below and next to my stove. This makes it easy for me to reach and grab while I'm cooking.**

- **COOKBOOKS: Don't waste prime location space on your cookbooks, especially if you make the same four meals each week. Store those books above and out of the way. Maybe keep your favorite one out and decoratively on display, for inspiration.**

- **KITCHEN TOWELS: I keep my towels in a non–prime location drawer but still handy in the kitchen. One towel always stays neatly on the handle of my oven, allowing me to grab it when I'm taking something out of the oven. I store a bunch of kitchen rags under my sink with the cleaning supplies. Rags are not to be confused with kitchen towels that are cute. I keep a special rag container handy with my cleaning supplies for cleaning up spills and messes my kids make. This avoids wasting my paper towels.**

- **TUPPERWARE: One of my favorite things! But keeping all the tops and bottoms together is a challenge. So I organize them in a cupboard near my sink, where they are** handy for storing leftovers, after we're done with dinner and cleaning up. I also have a separate, larger box for older, crappier Tupperware. This is for the Tupperware that is old or missing the lids. I'll take a random piece of Tupperware out of this box and throw my kids' crayons in them, or pour water, for their paintbrushes. Separating your Tupperware makes it easy to find the good stuff for storing food and grab the icky stuff for your kids' playtime things.

- **APPLIANCES:** Your countertops should only be adorned with the appliances you use on a regular basis, like a toaster oven, your coffeemaker, and a microwave. Random infomercial impulse buys *do not* get to live in that space! In your bottom cabinets, just below your cooking area, store frequently used appliances for easy access while you prep food.

- **CLEANING SUPPLIES:** I store all my cleaning supplies and things with chemicals under my sink. If you have little kids, this cabinet should have a childproof lock on it. I put the products I use most frequently toward the front. I also keep a bucket for rags and one for sponges. I have a small cupboard but I can still make it work.

KIDS' ROOM

Tackle your munchkins' messes the same way you would tackle yours: one spot at a time, making piles of items to toss, keep, and consider. If your kids have a hard time watching you sort or throw their stuff away, don't do it in front of them! Every item will become "special" and a "must-keep," and you'll be drowning in clutter. Just do it behind their backs and save yourself the headache!

Get rid of toys, clothes, accessories (one mitten? one pink sock?), video games, etc. Anything your kid has no interest in anymore—out it goes. Donate to a school, day-care center, or have a toy swap with the neighbors. I also allow each of my kids to have a "junk box" in their rooms. This is a privilege and is not to be abused! Almost everything in their rooms has a designated home: crayons go in the crayon box; Legos go in the Legos box; Barbies go in their home. The junk box is for all the "I don't know what"s. Anything from a random lip gloss or unlatching earrings to pieces of a Hot Wheels set or a favor from a classmate's birthday party go here. For my kids, it's a treasure trove, and they love digging in it. I just love having all their junk in one contained place!

GARAGE

If you can't park your car in your garage, it's time to de-clutter! Excess bikes and sporting equipment, tools, gardening supplies all need to be tackled. Once you have gone through and decided what to keep and what to toss, have a garage sale. In terms of storage, I recommend keeping like things together (all car products should go in one box; all sports stuff in another) and investing in some heavy-duty plastic containers (not flimsy cardboard boxes) that can hold a load. Most garages have abundant wall space, so consider hanging things up on hooks or even installing a rack or shelving system. The key is to get it all off the floor—that's where the clutter can happen. Just be warned: the garage is a big project. It can be dirty; it can be populated with little unexpected visitors (e.g., mice and bugs). But if you take it one corner at a time, you'll one day be proud to open your garage door and have people see inside!

cLEAN Momma Pop Quiz: Is It Time to De-clutter?

Ask yourself the following five questions:

1. Do you see clutter? In your drawers? On the floor? On your dresser tops?

2. Does it take a month to pick out an outfit? Can you easily find your favorite jeans or are they hiding behind an ugly pair of outdated palazzo pants?

3. Do you keep your clean laundry sitting in a pile for a week before you put it away?

4. Do you keep your dirty laundry piling up till you can smell it?

5. What's your bedtime routine? Do you read? Do you watch TV? Is your nightstand covered with remotes, magazines, and stacks of books?

If you answered YES to any of the above, you are more than in need of a cLEAN-up!

8
Calming Your Inner Chaos

cLEAN Momma Says . . . In this case, it's not "stuff" you're going to be ridding your life of. It's the mental blocks that are holding you back, making you feel "stuck" and sapping your strength, energy, and time.

YOUR CHAPTER 8 LAUNDRY LIST

- Examine your mind for clutter: what is building up and getting in your way?
- Acknowledge that fear, anger, and worry can hold you back—and learn how to redirect these emotions.
- Set your priorities and bring order to your obligations: you are allowed to say no and ask for help when you need it.

Just like your home, your mind can get filled to the brim with clutter. It's a feeling of being out of balance—for me, something akin to a chicken running around with her head cut off. I prefer to feel calm and in control—but that, like cleaning your home, takes time, effort, and a process of letting go.

Instead of evaluating your closets for "Do I need it? Can I use it?" you're going to look at your thoughts, feelings, and behaviors. Which ones are beneficial, which ones are making it difficult for you to make the right choices and move forward?

STOP PUTTING THINGS OFF. It may be one task or a dozen (these things do have a way of piling up, don't they?). Maybe you feel overwhelmed with obligations. What's holding you back? Is it a time commitment? Fear of failure? Make a list of what you think needs to be done. When you're clear on those tasks, you can make a plan and set a deadline for yourself. Choose one small thing to do and do it. Don't waste time deciding if it's the right thing to finish—just finish it. It will help you break out of your pattern of standing still.

WHY WORRY? It serves no purpose except to keep you from enjoying the present. When a worrying thought pops up, kick it out the door. Worry is a result of not having a plan of action. Focus your energy instead on the positive outcome—what you'd like to happen, instead of what you wish wouldn't happen.

LET GO OF ANGER. This is a biggie. I am a believer in "forgive and forget." Anger is bad for you both emotionally and physically. It's straining and draining and can make you do things impulsively that you'll later regret. Let go of grudges; move past petty arguments. Dwelling on them only makes you feel worse. Isn't it better to put the pain behind you?

TAKE A BREAK FROM NEGATIVITY. The world is filled with it, so is it any wonder your mind is, too? Spend one peaceful weekend (or just a day, if you can't afford two) without computers, phones, TV, magazines. No news is good news! Tune into your own positive channel. Spend the day in the beautiful sunshine, playing with your kids, soaking up the rays, breathing the clean air. Don't you just feel better thinking about it?

GET GOOD SLEEP. Allow your mind at least six to eight hours of downtime and R&R. It sounds so simple, but a good night's sleep can completely recharge your brain, making you less irritable, anxious, and out of sorts.

GO SLOWER. Think of yourself moving in slow motion instead of racing through life. Take things at a more leisurely pace: the way you walk, talk, move. This can do wonders to calm a harried brain as well!

VENT. Sometimes simply unburdening your load on a friend or family member can help you feel sane. Talk about what's bothering you, then, once you've gotten it out, don't allow those thoughts to creep back into your mind. When I am freakin' out, I call my friends or family. I like to call different people for different things. For example, my besties don't always understand work issues, while my mother and sisters do. Always ask first if you can share just to get it out. Let the other person know if you would like their help finding a solution or just a shoulder to lean on. Try not to abuse people's shoulders. Sometimes writing it out can be just as effective as venting. That being said, I can always count on my BFF Michelle to come over at two A.M., if I'm desperate, and hear me out!

Set Your Priorities

Bringing order to my obligations gives me a sense of instant calm and control. If I have a ton on my plate, the first thing I do is mentally sort that list into three categories: must do, should do, would be nice to do. The important thing is to recognize that you don't have to do them all at once. The situation isn't entirely overwhelming and hopeless. In fact, it's totally doable—if you prioritize.

Prioritizing is asking, "What's important to me?" When you answer that question, it becomes crystal-clear what you should be spending your time doing and what you should be focusing on. For me, it's all about quality over quantity. I learned that lesson when I went bankrupt. I was really able to prioritize what was important in my life. Taking care of my kids, doing things that will ensure they're safe, happy, and well-cared for—that's *numero uno*. And that's how I organize every day. What things need to be done that will help me achieve my top priority?

Once you know what needs to be done first, last, and always, consider your time constraints. Be honest with yourself: is this an attainable goal? If not, you'll wind up disappointed, pissed, and back in the same cluttered mess where you began. Smart prioritizers know how and when to delegate or ask for help. After dinner, I would always get up and immediately clear the table and do all the dishes. Then, midway through drying the pots and pans, I would get so frustrated and resentful that no one helped me. I felt like a maid. Why? Because I was behaving like one. Point being, if I wanted help, all I needed to do was nicely ask for assistance. Instead of nagging after the fact, I learned to simply say, "Would you mind helping me clear the table while I wash the dishes?" All of a sudden, I had helpers! And my family learned that everyone pitches in; everyone has a job to do.

It's also important to stop agonizing over each task you have to accomplish. This is perfectionism at its ugliest. You get so caught up in the details and spend so much time on one project, it prevents you from getting the rest of the things checked off your list. I am all for doing the very best job you can, but nobody—I repeat, nobody—is perfect. Sometimes you simply have to say, "Okay, this is the best I can do!" and move on.

cLEAN Momma Pop Quiz: Are You a Procrastinator?

Before you say "Nah! Not me!" answer the following questions truthfully. If you say YES to more than five, it's time to stop the avoidance act!

1. I always have to rush to finish a task.
2. I tend to put things off till "later" or "tomorrow."
3. If someone calls or e-mails, I don't get back to them right away.
4. My to-do list is usually a mile long.
5. I often feel guilty for not getting something done.
6. I start working on a big project a few days before it's due.
7. I'm often late to appointments.
8. I like "living on the edge."
9. I frequently forget friends' or family's birthdays and anniversaries.
10. If I have something difficult to tell someone, I avoid them like the plague!

Putting something off doesn't make it go away. Instead, tune out distractions, focus on what you can do (even if it's something small and minor), and don't allow yourself to constantly slip into crisis mode. Frazzled and frantic is not a good look on anyone.

9
cLEAN Momma on the Road

cLEAN Momma Says...
Taskercise has no boundaries. Don't
worry who might be watching...
just think how much hotter you'll
look when you're toned and taut!

YOUR CHAPTER 9 LAUNDRY LIST

- Practice Taskercise wherever and whenever.

- Find new, creative ways to sneak exercise into your life.

- Embrace the cLEAN Momma approach as a lifestyle commitment.

Now that you've familiarized yourself with the cLEAN Momma workout (and, hopefully, are doing those leg lifts as you scrub your counters!), it's time to hit the road. My clients are always coming up with new ways and places to Taskercise, and I *love* it. Get creative; you now know all the basics, so when and where can you employ them? How about . . .

Parked at your kids' school at pickup:
Carpool Crunches

1. While in the driver's seat, sit up tall with shoulders down and abs engaged. Put both hands on your steering wheel for support.

2. Lift your knees up toward the wheel and hold for 1 or 2 seconds, then lower them. (Make sure you don't touch the pedals.)

3. Repeat by bringing your knees up and down 10 times, then rest. Do this for at least 1 minute, or dare yourself to do this till your kids come out to the car, if you're early!

Cruising the aisles of the supermarket:
The Grab and Stretch

1. Stand with your feet hip-width apart.

2. As you reach for an item on the top shelf, stretch your arm.

3. Engage your tummy muscles and rise up on to your toes. Do this 10 times (unless there's someone in the aisle trying to get by you!).

In line at the deli counter: The Deli Belly

1. Stand in line with your hands on your grocery cart and your feet shoulder-width apart.

2. Slowly extend your cart out in front of you.

3. Focusing only on your ab muscles, use your tummy to bring your cart back toward you. This is very subtle, and the key is to not use your arms (bending your elbows) to bring your cart in and out, but rather to let your abs do all the work. Make sure you keep your shoulders down.

Filling your gas tank: Gas Squat

1. After you put the nozzle in your car's tank, stand with your feet shoulder-width apart and get into a deep squat, feet facing forward.

2. Use the side of your car for support but don't lean completely against it.

3. Your weight should be more on the heels of your feet as you sit back into the squat. This will help lift your tush rather than bulking up your thighs.

4. Hold till you finished filling, or for 30 seconds.

Cleaning your pool/yard: The Pool Pull

1. Stand with your feet shoulder-width apart and slightly bend your knees while you keep your tush tucked in.

2. Extend your arms out while you grab on to the net, collecting leaves out of the pool.

3. As you gather the leaves, keep your abs engaged. Bring the net or rake toward your body by using your abs more than your arms. Again, this is very subtle. It is about engaging your ab muscles and letting them do all the work.

In the playground: Svelte Swings

1. Stand with your feet shoulder-width apart and your knees slightly bent.

2. Engage your abs as you push your child.

3. Start with your right hand, and push your child 5 times. Make sure you don't twist your body and you really use your arms and abs to get in the push.

4. Switch to the left for 5 pushes. Alternate which hand pushes for as long as your kid wants to swing (that could be hours, I warn you!).

In the air: Airplane Abs

1. Sit back in your airplane seat. Rest your arms and hands on the armrests.

2. Contract your abs and tuck your tush in, making your torso into a "C" curve.

3. Slowly raise both feet off the floor several inches.

4. Hold your feet in the air for 1 second before you bring them back to the floor. (Don't put your feet entirely on the floor; gently tap your toes.)

5. Bring them up and down 10–15 times, then rest, and repeat.

6. To kick it up a notch, on your last one, pulse your knees in the air an extra 10–15 times.

In the air: Airplane Arm Stretch

1. Sit in your airplane seat and scoot your tush a bit forward.

2. Place both hands on the armrests and sit up tall with your spine straight and shoulders down.

3. Keep your hands on the armrests and try to touch your elbows together behind you. Really squeeze your back muscles together and stretch your chest muscles in front. You can also drop and relax your neck for an added stretch. Make sure you keep your shoulders down the entire time.

In a hotel: The Hotel Hot Wall Squat

1. Stand tall with your abs engaged, your shoulders down, and your back against a wall, placing your feet about two feet out in front of you. Your feet should be hip-width apart.

2. Bending your knees, slide your back down the wall until your knees are at a ninety-degree angle. Make sure your knees are directly over your ankles; you may need to inch your feet farther from the wall to create the proper alignment. Your thighs should remain parallel to the floor.

3. Hold for 30–60 seconds, and then stand up. Repeat for a total of 3 reps.

4. To kick it up a notch, alternate between lifting your left heel for a few seconds and then your right one.

Variation: Hot Wall Squat with Knees

1. Stand tall with your abs engaged, your shoulders down, and your back against a wall, placing your feet about two feet out in front of you. Your feet should be hip-width apart.

2. Bending your knees, slide your back down the wall until your knees are at a ninety-degree angle. Make sure your knees are directly over your ankles; you may need to inch your feet farther from the wall to create the proper alignment. Your thighs should remain parallel to the floor.

3. Hold this position while you squeeze your knees in and out together 10–15 times, rest, and repeat. The key to this exercise is to really keep your spine straight and your tush in as much as possible, curving the small of your back under you. As you squeeze your knees together, also squeeze your inner thighs.

4. To kick this up a notch, rise up onto the balls of your feet for the entire set of 10–15.

In a hotel: Hotel Stair Cardio

The truth is, even when I'm on vacation (shoving all-you-can-eat buffet food into my big mouth), I still want to get my heart rate up, and sweat. That said, I'm not paying twenty bucks to use the hotel spa to run on a treadmill for forty-five minutes when I have stairwells at the end of every hallway calling my name!

1. Go to a stairwell and head to the bottom floor of the hotel.

2. Climb up the first set of stairs and then power walk or jog to the end of the hall and climb the other flight of stairs.

3. Walk up one flight and exit, power walk or jog back to the other end of the hall, and go up *that* flight of stairs.

4. Repeat till you make your way to the roof.

5. When you get to the top, stretch for 1 minute, then start your way back down to the bottom and repeat.

6. Do this for 30 minutes, no matter how many floors there are. You can always take the elevator if you start to pass out! Remember to pace yourself and start slowly, working your way up to a fast speed!

cLEAN Eating on the Road

Just because you're not home or in your neighborhood, doesn't mean it's time to go back to your bad habits. It's always possible to make healthy choices *anywhere*—even at a truck stop or a 7-Eleven.

At a Mexican joint

- Chose a protein plate of chicken, veggies, and black beans and go for bust on the salsa, you can never have too much!

- Black bean soup or tortilla soup is better to fill up on than a basket of chips. Plus, you'll feel less inclined to dig into the burrito grande.

At a Chinese/sushi place

- Order the miso soup or wonton soup first. Tons of veggies and the broth is super-filling.

- Avoid the rice and noodle dishes. Better to have shrimp or chicken in a spicy brown sauce and pile it with the veggies!

- Instead of sushi rolls filled with rice, try sashimi (plain fish) with rice served on the side.

At a pizza restaurant

- Always think thin! Deep dish is deep trouble, especially on the thighs. Order thin crust.

- If you can swap veggies for pepperoni, even better!

- An easy trick to avoid eating the entire pie is to have a side salad with light dressing before you indulge in the pizza.

At a fast-food burger chain

- Order a grilled chicken breast, or a kids' burger if you have to eat one. Ask for extra lettuce/tomato and remove half the bun, so it's open-faced.

- If you have to have fries, order the kid-size portion and only eat half.

- A snack wrap with extra lettuce and tomato is another option: look for grilled chicken options and order sans dressing and cheese.

In a convenience store or airport

- Buy a cup of yogurt, string cheese, almonds, hard-boiled eggs, or bananas. Tons of options besides the Slurpee machine!

cLEAN Momma Pop Quiz: Do You Make cLEAN Choices on the Road?

It's so easy to say, "Well, I'm on vacation . . . ," and throw away your good habits and hard work for junk food. Be honest and answer the following statements true or false:

_____ If I'm on a road trip, it's okay to hit 7-Eleven.

_____ If I'm in a hotel room, the vending machine is my best friend at night.

_____ Airports are a good excuse to eat Auntie Anne's pretzels, Micky D's, and Häagen-Dazs . . . because airplane food is terrible!

_____ I can have a caramel macchiato. It's just coffee.

_____ I can have three piña coladas at the pool. What's wrong? It's fruit!

If you answered TRUE to any of the above, you are in denial! So have your three cocktails and enjoy them, have your Big Mac if you want it—just be aware of what you're putting in your body and that there are smarter choices you can make.

10
cLEAN Family

cLEAN Momma Says . . . Teach your kids by example how to live happy and healthy lives.

YOUR CHAPTER 10 LAUNDRY LIST

- Introduce your kids to cLEAN living by making it fun and tasty!
- Learn ways to Taskercise while you spend quality time with your kids.
- Teach your children why it's important to eat healthy and mindfully—the routines they develop today can last a lifetime.

The best part about having cLEAN Momma for a momma? My kids get to hear and see me do my cLEAN routine every day. Although, if you ask them:

"My mommy cleans stuff and it's really boring!"—Jack
"My mommy looks like a dork when she cleans!"—Sophie

Dork or no dork, I am glad that my kids see me in action. I'm setting an example. I never refer to foods as "good" or "bad." Instead, we talk about "growing foods" or "healthy foods." You don't want to give food any more power than it already has! I try to introduce something new to my kids by eating it first. They get curious . . . they might smell it or take a nibble. And if they don't like it, fine. I'll never force it: you don't want to turn mealtime into a showdown. If at first you don't succeed with the squash and snow peas, try, try again another time.

I give my kids a lot of credit: they're not stupid. They know when their mom is trying to put one over on them. I can't bury broccoli under mac 'n' cheese. Instead, I treat them with respect and give them the same tools that I would use: awareness, moderation, open-mindedness. I want them to understand *why* we eat what we do. How food is fuel and energy, not just something we gulp down in between episodes of *iCarly* and *SpongeBob*. A few more ways to get your gang eating healthy:

SHOW, DON'T TELL. Children will naturally mirror what they see. So, if you practice good, healthy habits, they'll follow your lead. If you grab fast food for lunch, of course they're going to want it, too! Remember you're setting a good example, and reach for healthy choices.

"IT'S YOUR CHOICE." If I tell my kids, "You can't have it," they will undoubtedly whine, beg, or nag me until I give it to them. So instead, I use this approach:

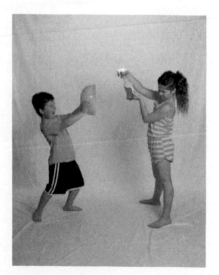

THEM: "Mommy, can we have a KitKat?"

ME: "You can have that if you really want it . . . it's your choice. But I have to say, having some apples with peanut butter is a healthier option. It's up to you."

They automatically go for the KitKat. Pause.

THEM: "Is this good for me?"

ME: "No, not really. But have it if you want. It's your body."

THEM: "Well, maybe we'll have just a little . . ."

ME: "Then have a little."

Pause. Silence. They huddle in the corner.

THEM: "Mommy, can we have some apple and peanut butter?"

If we force anything, it creates resistance. So instead, let's educate our kids and allow them to decide.

GET THEM COOKIN'. Even the pickiest of eaters will try new foods if you let them loose in the kitchen. I like to let my kids cook with me: we chop, mix, and toss together, and they're eager to eat whatever dish (no matter how healthy!) they've helped to prepare. It's also a great chance to spend some good quality time with your kid while you get the meal under way.

AROUND THE WORLD IN EIGHTY DISHES. Here's a fun way to get your child excited about sampling something. Pretend you're going on a trip to someplace far away: India, France, Hawaii. Talk about what you'd find there—what sights, smells, and exotic foods. Then serve something for lunch or dinner that includes one of those foods. You can even teach your child a few words of the language (like "please" and "thank you") and try it out at the table.

EAT TOGETHER. That means sitting down at a table, having a meal and a conversation as a family. Be present. Sure, it might be easier to eat standing up or on the run, but you need to let your child see you in eating action (that role-model thing again). I also feel that when we're talking about school or the day, my kids are distracted and will eat just about anything on their plates. Also, set some ground rules for all of you: no TV, no computer, and no texting during dinnertime.

Playtime Taskercise

I am a hands-on mommy who loves to spend quality time with my kids. We get on the floor and dress Barbies or build Legos, chat about school and friends, watch Disney Channel shows, and read *Green Eggs and Ham*. But I've also found a way to sneak in my workout when I'm with them. It's a win-win; I do for them while I do for me.

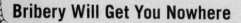

Bribery Will Get You Nowhere

Your kid is having a major tantrum in the frozen-food aisle and you see a solution on the horizon: Ben & Jerry's. So you plead, "Please, just be quiet and Mommy will give you a treat!" The tears and tantrum instantly subside as your kid pops the Popsicle in his mouth. Or maybe your kiddies refuse to touch the pile of peas you've put on their plates. So you say, "Eat them all and you can have dessert!" Every mom knows better, yet every mom does it. Why? Because bribing kids with sweets will (a) get them to do whatever you want and (b) get them to shut the hell up when your nerves are as raw as the meat at the butcher's counter. I get it. If you choose to have a reward system in your home, try a sticker or a small toy instead of a lolly. Otherwise, you're teaching your child that food is a reward and a coping mechanism. You'll be raising tomorrow's emotional eater.

THE PRETEND BIKE

WHAT YOU NEED: A comfy rug, carpeted floor, or a yoga mat

WHERE YOU DO IT: Living room, playroom, kids' room

WHAT IT WORKS: Lower abs, obliques, and core

1. Lie face-up on the floor. Place your hands behind your head, lightly supporting it with your fingers.

2. Bring your knees in to your chest and lift your shoulder blades off the floor without pulling on your neck.

3. Rotate to the left, bringing your right elbow toward your left knee as you straighten the other leg.

4. Switch sides, bringing your left elbow toward your right knee.

5. Continue alternating sides, "pedaling" for one to three sets of 12–16 reps until the commercial break's over or your kids jump on top of you!

PLAYTIME CRUNCH

WHAT YOU NEED: A comfy rug, carpeted floor, towel, or a yoga mat

WHERE YOU DO IT: Living room, playroom, kids' room

WHAT IT WORKS: Waist, abs, and "muffin top"

1. Lie on your back with your legs straight up, then crisscross your knees.

2. Place your hands behind your head for support, but don't pull on your neck.

3. Tighten your tummy, imagining your belly button being drawn down toward your spine.

4. Lift your shoulder blades off the floor, like you're reaching your chest toward your feet.

5. Keep the legs steady in this position and really focus on your belly button sucking in toward your spine at the top of the movement.

6. Lower and repeat for one to three sets of 12–16 reps, or in between playing Legos and board games.

SNOW ANGELS

WHAT YOU NEED: A comfy rug, carpeted floor, towel, or a yoga mat

WHERE YOU DO IT: Living room, playroom, kids' room

WHAT IT WORKS: Core, thighs

1. Lie flat on your back with your legs out in front of you and your arms to your sides, palms facing your body.

2. Think of your belly button touching your spine. This will help flatten the small of your back. Inhale through your nose.

3. As you exhale, lift your shoulders and legs off the floor about four inches.

4. On the inhale, bring your arms out to the side and your legs as well. (This looks like a snow angel.)

5. Bring your legs back together as well as your arms to your sides.

6. Bring your legs and arms in and out 10 times while keeping your shoulders and arms up the entire time.

DONKEY KICK-OUTS

WHAT YOU NEED: A low table (such as a coffee table) for support

WHERE YOU DO IT: Living room, playroom, kids' room

WHAT IT WORKS: Core, tush, and legs

1. Kneel down. Place your elbows on your coffee table for support.

2. Keeping your shoulders and hips square to the table, lean slightly forward. Slowly kick your right leg in the air behind you. Fully extend the leg up as high as you can.

3. Bend your knee and kick out in a forty-five-degree angle. Repeat 10–15 times on each leg.

If you keep your foot flexed and your abs tight, you'll work your tush hard, as well as your core!

PLAY TIME, TUSH TIME

WHAT YOU NEED: A comfy rug, carpeted floor, or a yoga mat

WHERE YOU DO IT: Living room, playroom, kids' room

WHAT IT WORKS: Waist and core

1. Lie on the floor and place your hands on the floor or behind your head.

2. Bring your knees in toward your chest until they're bent to ninety degrees, with your feet together or crossed.

3. Suck in your tummy to curl your hips off the floor, reaching your legs up toward the ceiling.

4. It's a very small movement, so try to use your abs to lift your hips rather than swinging your legs and creating momentum.

5. Lower and repeat for one to three sets of 12–16 reps, on until your kids jump on top of you, yelling "MOMMY, MOMMY, MOMMY!"

PLANK OUT

WHAT YOU NEED: A comfy rug, carpeted floor, or a yoga mat

WHERE YOU DO IT: Living room, playroom, kids' room

WHAT IT WORKS: Arms, shoulders, core

1. Lie facedown on the floor. (Put a towel down, or a mat, 'cause *eww*). Rest on your forearms, palms flat on the floor.

2. Push off the floor, rising up on to your toes and resting on your elbows. (It's pretty hard, so make sure you do this with proper form!)

3. Keep your back flat, in a straight line from your head to your heels, and your neck in line with your spine.

4. Tuck your tush under and suck in your tummy. Remember to breathe and be sure not to stick your tush in the air or sag down in the middle!

5. Hold for 20–60 seconds, lower, and repeat 3–5 times.

THE COBRA

WHAT YOU NEED: A space to stand tall

WHERE TO DO IT: Anywhere you have the room

WHAT IT WORKS: Borrowed from yoga, this pose will strengthen your neck and your back, as you meditate through the chaos around you. My kids laugh at me when I do this one.

1. Stand tall with your feet shoulder-width apart, shoulders down, and arms by your sides.

2. Extend your head back and squeeze your shoulder blades together.

3. Breathe in through your nose. Hold for 30 seconds. Breathe out through the mouth.

cLEAN Eating for Kiddies

The eating habits your kids pick up from you when they're young will help them maintain a healthy lifestyle when they are adults. That said, I don't believe in being a dictator; I don't force-feed my children veggies and I don't ban junk entirely. They're kids! What's fun about being a kid if you can't eat crap now and then? Instead, I try to educate and empower them. This is what's healthy, and this is what you can choose. The power is in your hands. Most of the time, they make the smart choice. Sometimes they pick the KitKat. What are you gonna do? But when I cook for my kids, I try to make the meals both fun and nutritious. I have to say, my kids actually enjoy eating healthy food.

FROZEN SMOOTHIE POPPERS

My kids love this tasty treat! Smoothies are yummy but frozen smoothie poppers, now we're talkin'!

Blend 1 cup fresh strawberries or blueberries, ¼ cup apple juice, ½ cup pineapple juice, and some ice. Then pour it into an ice cube tray. Cover the tray with plastic wrap. Poke toothpicks through the wrap to make mini popsicle sticks. Freeze overnight.

EGG IN A MUG

This is super-easy, convenient, and a great mid-day snack or breakfast.

Get a mug and 2 eggs. Use 1 yolk and 2 egg whites. Swish it up in your mug, adding 1 tsp. low-fat cream cheese. Microwave for 1½ minutes till it's fluffy. Add salt and pepper to taste. You can also throw in ¼ cup chopped spinach or mushrooms.

FIVE-MINUTE LEMON CHICKEN

I swear this takes just 5 minutes to prep! It's easy and fast for a school night, and my family loves it.

Take a few chicken breasts or drumsticks (kids like these, because they can hold them). Spread them out in a baking dish, either skinless (less fat) or with the skin. Use about 4 lemons and squeeze the juice all over. Cut up some fresh garlic (about 1 clove) and sprinkle over the chicken. Sprinkle with salt and pepper and drizzle with olive oil (about 2 Tbsp.) on top. Bake at 400°F for 45 minutes, until the chicken is crispy on the outside and juicy inside.

MINI PIZZA BREADS

Kids love cute finger food!

Spread some tomato sauce on a slice of whole-wheat or whole-grain bread and sprinkle cheese (shredded low-fat mozzarella) on top. You can add mushrooms, veggies, or olives for an extra nutritional punch. Bake on 350°F for 10 minutes till the cheese is melted and toast is a bit crispy. I like to cut them into four squares, then diagonally again, to form mini-triangles.

BAKED BROCCOLI CRISPS

Whenever my kids are craving a salty, greasy sensation (aka potato chips), I bake up these delicious crisps.

Cut broccoli into small niblets and spread on a greased cookie sheet. Drizzle 2 Tbsp. olive oil over the top and sprinkle with salt. Bake at 400°F for about 25 minutes. It should come out crispy and crunchy and finger-lickin' good!

cLEAN Momma Pop Quiz: Are You Setting the Right Example for Your Kids?

You always want to teach your children by example; they will mirror you. But are you aware of your behaviors? Answer TRUE or FALSE to the following:

_____ I scold my kid for throwing her clothes on the floor . . . but I can't walk into my walk-in closet.

_____ I encourage my child to eat healthy snacks . . . but I grab a candy bar when I'm starving.

_____ I tell my child it's great to be active. . . . but I haven't worked out in a month.

_____ I try to serve my child the right-size portions . . . but if that pizza is good, I'll finish the whole pie when he's sleeping.

_____ I tell my kids to stay away from sugary soft drinks . . . but I order a soda and drink it in front of them, saying, "This isn't good for you, but I'm a grown-up."

If you answered TRUE to any of the above, you are normal! Just be honest with yourself and your kids, and own it.

Staying cLEAN

YOU DID IT. YOU CLEANED up your life top to bottom. You have a new approach to living, eating, and exercising, every day. You feel stronger, saner, more able to cope with whatever crap lands in your lap. Applause, applause! But now comes the tough part: sticking to it. How do you maintain this new lifestyle?

First off, it takes **PLANNING**. As I have learned the hard way, you can't just leave it to chance. You can't stick your head in the sand—or up your butt! The crazier your week, the more you can plan ahead. You now have the tools. You have charts and how-tos and recipes. Stay organized; stay on track. If you get overwhelmed, take a breath and step back. Look at the big picture. When all else fails, go back to home base: chapter 1, where you learned how to be present and focused on the here and now. Write stuff down ('cause god knows, I'd forget my head if it wasn't pinned to my shoulders!), and make a plan of action.

Remember that you always (unless there is a gun pointing to your head) have a **CHOICE**. You can choose to have a salad for lunch or a Fatburger. You can choose to work out or lie on the couch eating Doritos. You can choose to stay stuck or you can choose to move forward. Choice is your greatest gift and greatest power.

Stay focused on the **POSITIVE**. Don't let that old self-doubt creep back in. You can do it. You are worthy. I don't ever want to see you in sloppy sweats again (unless you're working out!).

My mom always says, "Life is a journey, good and bad." Translation: if we don't experience the crap, we don't appreciate the good! Enjoy the process of **SELF-GROWTH**. Instead of getting sucked into the poor-me pity party that keeps one stuck, focus on the big picture. Allow yourself to have your feelings. They're normal, and they'll help guide you, so listen to them. Change is a bitch—but going backward is worse!

START SMALL so you don't burn out. Having a plan of action and setting realistic goals makes us feel enthusiastic! You can't move forward if you are moving in circles. Stop repeating yourself, and shift! Taking chances can lead to failures, but that's okay; that's how we learn and grow. Failures are great lessons. Embrace your opportunities! They are right in front of you.

You just need to take the Windex out and wipe off your glasses!

ACKNOWLEDGMENTS

THANK YOU TO ALL THOSE who have a part in this journey . . . my life.

First and foremost, to my kids! My nine-year-old daughter keeps me real, honest, and accountable. Sophie, I think you are an amazing person. I'm proud of who you are, and I adore you. You are wise beyond your years and fantastically funny.

Jack, my six-year-old son, is kind, bright, loving, funny, and outrageous. He says the most random—often inappropriate—things to strangers, like "Hey, lady, are you gonna keep yappin'? We're watching a movie here." (That's when I hide.)

To my mother, aka "Waka Waka" or "Gramacha." Mom, you have been an inspiration to me. Your wisdom, tenacity, and enthusiasm for life have finally gotten through to me—and how beautiful that you finally get me "before you're dead," Sumitomo. I love you.

To Leslie, my other mommy: You have been so important in my life. You are nurturing, loving, and a strength and support I am grateful for. I love you. How very lucky I am to have you.

To my dad, "Aboo," who is, well, unconditionally there for me, I love you and feel so lucky to call you Dad.

To Steve, "Bug," who shares the ability to rise above the chaos and see the big picture, our kids. Friends since fifteen, friends for life. There's something wrong with the counterweights. xoxo Bug!

To my sisters, Deb and Amy, who inspired me to blog and helped me get the ball rolling, who listen to my problems, and who are there for me no matter what. I love you.

To Llama, Stephanie Holt-Lecovin, who has been "the wind beneath my wings." You have been an inspiration and a true best friend, since the days of Barbies in the lake, "poppers," and *Divorce Court* with Oreos. I truly thank you for being my friend for life, my inspiration, and an amazing part of this book.

To Geoff Lecovin, who takes good care of my llama. I thank you for your help!

To Bubbie. I will always go to Neil Diamond concerts with you, as long as you promise not to drive so we end up lost and at a Barry Manilow concert instead. I love you, but you know that!

To Michelle, my wife. I love your shoes and despise doing the dishes at your house. Thank you for your amazing ability to always be inside my brain . . . enough said. xo

To Laura, *Mi Gallo se murio ayer.* I just felt like being random for you. I'm amazed by you, and I love you.

To Shmack, Advil is meant for headaches, wine is great for anxiety, and kale tastes like crap. (Just kidding, you hot lady!) I'm proud of you. I love you, and I adore you.

To Dave, tenacity defines you. May we all remember to smell the pines.

To Miata, who knew we would take Kiera and Sophie to *Annie* one day? You impress me, and I admire and respect who you are.

To Sarma and Larry Rosenberg, my first and most amazing dance teachers. To "Morty."

To those who helped with my DVD, I truly thank you: Vanessa Ruanne, Steve Lang, Fernando, Mike Garcia, Todd Green, and Dean Kramer.

To Jim Byrnes, who was there from the beginning, I thank you. To Robin Doyle, my girlfriend/press agent, who sent out my first press release. (Who knew?)

To Alyia Silverstein, you are truly amazing!

To Paul Fedorko, my agent, who is beyond super-awesome and cool! And to Sammy Bina. To Sid Kaufman, my agent, a man of many words . . . six words for you: You're fantastic, and I thank you.

To Bob Hagarty, who wrote a wonderful article in the *Wall Street Journal*, I thank you. Truly. To Michael Morrison, who read the article. To HarperCollins, including everyone in design, production, publicity, and marketing for a truly amazing opportunity to share my big, fat mouth. I have a lot to say.

To Lisa Sharkey, huge thanks!

To Amy, for being a great editor. Have a great birth. Take drugs!

And to Sheryl Berk, who brilliantly helped me spit my thoughts onto paper, I'm so grateful to you. I think you are truly amazing!